The Essential Guide to

Bowel Cancer

IAN EUSTACE

Published in Great Britain in 2018 by
need2know
Remus House
Coltsfoot Drive
Peterborough
PE2 9BF
Telephone 01733 898103
www.need2knowbooks.co.uk

Contents

Introduction

The word "cancer" can provoke stronger emotions than almost any other word in the English language, but we can't possibly know what cancer actually means for our families, our friends, our future and ourselves without the proper information. By now, many cancers can be cured, early diagnosis is far more possible and treatments are constantly improving, because we actually know quite a lot about the illness.

Here are some facts about bowel cancer:

- Bowel cancer tends to develop in older people – about 80% of cases are diagnosed in people 60 or above.

- Most people don't have cancer, even if their symptoms look a lot like bowel cancer. The symptoms of bowel cancer are shared with many other conditions that are far less serious, such as hemorrhoids (piles).

- Bowel cancer does not appear to be on the increase, diagnosis is being made earlier through screening programmes, and treatment is getting better.

- The third most common cancer, more than 37,000 people experience bowel cancer each year in the UK alone.

- It's possible to manage bowel cancer effectively, allowing you to live your life as normal for a long time.

This book is aimed at reassuring those of us who are worried that they might have cancer but, in fact, screening programmes and clinical studies tell us that in most cases, cancer is not the cause of their symptoms. For healthy individuals it also gives valuable information about what you can do to reduce the risk of developing bowel cancer and gives useful tips on healthy eating and lifestyle.

The goal of this book is to provide anyone interested in learning about bowel cancer with the information they need. The book has also been written to help people who have been diagnosed with bowel cancer, as well as their friends and family, to understand symptoms, treatments, causes and potential outcomes of bowel cancer. Many other conditions that are far less serious than bowel cancer share its symptoms, and this is important to keep in mind.

This book also contains advice on how to cope with cancer on a daily basis if you have been diagnosed, along with practical information about your treatment choices.

A Note to the Reader

You should see your GP for individual medical advice about treatment of bowel cancer or any worries or concerns you might have. Professional medical advice should not be replaced by this book, which was written to give you general information only. The help list displays the many resources which provided the factual information in this book. For further information please refer to these resources. We have tried to keep the facts and figures as up-to-date as we possibly can.

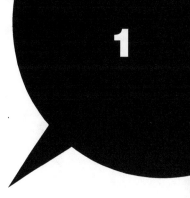

Bowel Cancer – What Does it Mean?

Talking about your bowels or going to the toilet can be very embarrassing and it may be hard to ask questions, however with the right information it should be easier to discuss this sensitive subject with your doctor. It's very important to have accurate information about this disease, as the word "cancer" can evoke a wide range of responses and feelings.

The help list at the end of the book gives information on where to access help and support. Whether it's prevention or treatment, this book should prepare you for anything you may have to deal with. We're starting with the basics in this chapter. More information and greater detail can be found in later chapters.

What Are Bowels?

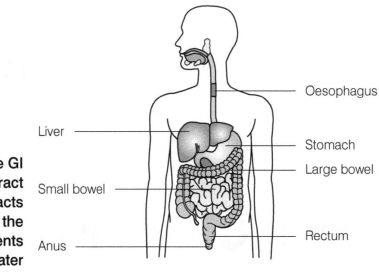

Oesophagus

Liver

Stomach

Large bowel

Small bowel

Rectum

Anus

The GI tract extracts all of the nutrients and water from the food we eat that our bodies need.

Your bowel is part of your GI (gastrointestinal) tract. The GI tract extracts all of the nutrients and water from the food we eat that our bodies need. The GI tract is also known as the digestive system, and consists of the rectum and colon (large bowel), small intestine (small bowel), stomach, oesophagus (gullet or food pipe) and mouth. Your food is digested and passed into the small bowel after it's transported from your mouth to your stomach. Essential nutrients are extracted from the food at this point. It's then passed out of the body through the back passage (rectum) via the anus, having had all of its water removed in the large bowel.

The Large Bowel

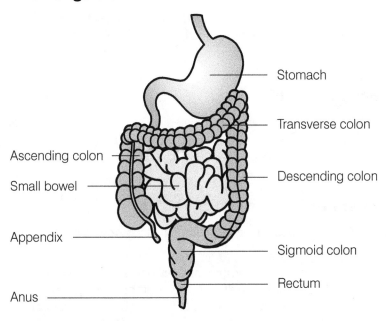

The small and large bowel are surrounded by a sheet of tissue known as the mesentery, which contains blood vessels that supply blood to the bowel and lymph nodes that drain away tissue fluid from the rectum. Consisting of the rectum and colon, the large bowel is the final section of your GI tract. It runs up the right side of your abdomen (trunk), beginning where it joins to the small bowel (next to the appendix).

This section is called the *ascending colon*. The *transverse colon* is the name for the section that crosses the body below the stomach, and is followed by the *descending colon* where it travels back down the left side of the abdomen. The *sigmoid colon*, an s-shaped bend, connects the descending colon to the rectum, which then leads to the external opening of the bowel – the anus. In total, the colon is about five feet long and has five distinct sections.

Small Bowels

The part of your GI tract immediately after the stomach is your small bowel. It's the longest section of the GI tract (about 20 feet in total), but is called the small bowel because it's thinner than the large bowel.

What Is Bowel Cancer?

"Bowel cancer" usually describes a cancer that originated in the rectum or colon (large bowel). The term "colorectal cancer" may also be used by your doctor. The cancer growth is usually called a tumour. Although it's extremely rare, cancer can also occur in the small bowel.

Types of bowel cancer

Bowel cancer is classified according to the type of tissue that it develops in. There are five different types.

- Adenocarcinoma: These tumours begin in the gland cells (cells that produce mucus to help move the stool through the bowel) of the bowel lining. This type of bowel cancer is the most common. It makes up over 95% of all bowel cancer cases. Depending on how the cells appear under the microscope, adenocarcinomas can be either signet ring or mucinous. Signet ring tumours consist of cells that contain mucus which pushes the nucleus to one side of the cell, giving it a signet ring-like appearance. Pools of mucus contain the cancer cells in mucinous tumours.

- Carcinoid tumours: These are rare types of neuroendocrine tumour, meaning that they develop in organs or tissues that produce hormones, usually in the GI tract. Around 2-7% of carcinoid tumours begin in the large bowel, 4-17% in the rectum.

- Lymphomas: Only about 1% of bowel cancers are lymphomas, tumours that begin in the lymphatic system.

- Sarcomas: These are tumours of the supporting cells of the body, such as muscle and bone. Leiomyosarcomas are sarcomas that form in the muscle of the bowel.

- Squamous cell carcinoma: Unlike gland cells, squamous cells do not produce mucus and are similar to skin cells. These tumours begin in the cells lining the bowel.

Risk Factors for Bowel Cancer

While some risk factors cannot be altered (non-modifiable), some are modifiable (can be altered) to increase or decrease your level of risk. Age and family history are examples of non-modifiable risk factors; in other words these are risk factors that you cannot change. Diet and lifestyle are two examples of modifiable risk factors. You can improve your lifestyle by exercising and maintaining a healthy weight, and change your diet to include healthier foods.

Family history

Risk is also increased by a family history of bowel cancer, especially if two close relatives (brother, sister, child or parent) are diagnosed with the condition or if one close relative is diagnosed before the age of 45.

How old are you?

More than 80% of bowel cancer cases are diagnosed in people over the age of 60. Age is the biggest risk factor for bowel cancer.

Chronic diseases of the bowel

The risk of bowel cancer can also be increased by long-lasting (chronic) diseases of the bowel.

The lining of the colon can experience open sores (ulcers), irritation and swelling in people with ulcerative colitis, a type of IBD (inflammatory bowel disease). Approximately 1% of bowel cancers develop as a result of ulcerative colitis. The cause is not known although there are links to genetics and a diet low in fibre. The condition can cause people to have bouts of diarrhoea which last for weeks, containing blood from any number of ulcers. People who have had ulcerative colitis for ten or more years in the bend between the transverse and descending parts of the colon (splenic flexure) have an increased risk of bowel cancer.

People with Crohn's disease have about a two and a half-fold increased risk of getting bowel cancer. About half of the people with Crohn's disease have inflammation and ulcers in both the small and large bowel, while about 20% have Crohn's just in the large bowel. Crohn's disease can affect the entire GI tract from the mouth to the anus and, like ulcerative colitis, is an inflammatory bowel disease. Severe episodes cause repeated damage to the bowel lining, with the condition causing chronic inflammation to the bowel.

Genetic factors

The risk of bowel cancer can also be increased by some inherited conditions. Your risk of developing a number of types of cancer – including bowel cancer – is increased if you have the rare genetic condition HNPCC (hereditary non-polyposis colorectal cancer, or Lynch syndrome). People with Lynch syndrome have a fault (or mutation) in the HNPCC gene which results in a lifetime risk of developing colon cancer of about 80%. This is a gene involved in our body's repair of DNA. Cancer of the lining of the womb or uterus, or endometrial cancer, is also increased to 80% risk in women with Lynch syndrome.

The growth of numerous polyps in the large bowel can be caused by FAP (familial adenomatous polyposis). FAP is very rare with only one in 7,000 people (less than 1%) with bowel cancer having the condition. The risk of getting bowel cancer is higher in people with FAP because of the number of polyps, and most will develop bowel cancer by age 40-50. Some can develop into cancer with time, but the majority will be benign (non-cancerous). To reduce the risk of bowel cancer, many people with FAP have surgery at the age of 25 ro remove the entire colon – this is known as a colectomy.

Turcot syndrome affects the same genes involved with Lynch syndrome and FAP. Similar to Lynch syndrome and FAP, Turcot syndrome is a condition associated with the formation of polyps in the bowel and faulty DNA repair leading to gene mutation. However, FAP and Lynch syndrome are far more common – Turcot syndrome is very rare.

Diabetes

We don't know why just yet, but it seems that people with diabetes have an increased likelihood of developing bowel cancer. Bowel cancer and type 2 diabetes (people who are not dependent on insulin injections) do share a number of risk factors, such as obesity, but people with type 2 diabetes still have an increased risk and often a poorer outcome post-diagnosis when these factors are taken into account.

Ethnicity

An increased risk of bowel cancer (around two to three times that of the general population) affects Ashkenazi Jewish people of Eastern European descent. This is thought to be a result of a mutation of the APC (adenomatous polyposis coli) gene called I1307K, and goes some way towards explaining why the most common cause of cancer deaths in Israel is colorectal cancer. A mutated APC gene actually causes the cancer to grow rather than helping to prevent it, and is present in about 10% of Ashkenazi Jews.

Smoking

You have a higher risk of developing bowel cancer – as well as many other types of cancer (especially lung cancer) – if you smoke. Those who have never smoked have a much lower risk than current smokers, and even ex-smokers.

You are what you eat

An increased risk of bowel cancer has been linked to the consumption of certain foods. For example, the risk of bowel cancer is increased if an individual eats a large amount of processed and red meats. Certain types of fat, especially saturated fat (found in red meat and dairy products such as butter and cheese) and trans-fats (found in processed food) are thought to be linked to the formation of polyps.

Processed meat is treated to preserve it using methods such as curing, smoking, salting, or adding chemicals, and it is thought that these processes can result in the formation of carcinogens (cancer-causing chemicals). Cancer risk may be increased as a result of certain chemicals that are present in red meat. Damage to the lining of the colon may be caused by a substance called haem, which gives meat its red colour. It's also thought that chemicals that can cause bowel cancer may be produced when meat is cooked at a high temperature, such as by frying or roasting.

Fibre increases intestinal transit (the speed at which food moves through the bowel) and ensures that your bowel movements are regular. Risk of bowel cancer is also increased in those whose diets are low in fibre, which is a plant-based food also known as roughage. Potentially harmful chemicals are in contact with the cells lining the bowel for longer if you're not getting enough fibre, as your intestinal transit will be slowed down. To highlight the importance of fibre in the diet, traditional native Japanese people have a diet that is naturally high in fibre and they have a lower risk of bowel cancer compared to those living in Western Europe. Those who migrate to the West have the same risk of getting bowel cancer as Western people if they take up a Western-style diet. Their risk of bowel cancer increases when they change their diet from high fibre to low fibre. Constipation, where the stools become harder and more difficult to pass, can also occur as a result of low fibre diets.

You have a higher risk of developing bowel cancer – as well as many other types of cancer (especially lung cancer) – if you smoke.

Lifestyle

People who do not exercise appear to have poorer intestinal transit compared with people who exercise regularly. An increased risk of developing bowel cancer appears to be associated with obesity and low physical activity. Potentially harmful chemicals have a higher chance of being exposed to the cells of the bowel the longer food remains in the gut.

The relationships between cancer and lifestyle, environment, nutritional status and diet are being explored by a large European study of more than 500,000 people. This is the EPIC (European Prospective Investigation into Cancer and Nutrition) Study. So far, the observations of other studies that there are strong links between low physical activity, obesity and increased risk of bowel cancer have been supported by the study's key findings.

There is also a strong link between lack of exercise and weight gain, as those people who do not exercise do not use up enough energy to maintain a healthy weight. Healthy individuals have a BMI of less than 25; those who are overweight have a BMI of between 25 and 30, whilst obesity is associated with a BMI of more than 30. The Body Mass Index (BMI) is the tool used to measure obesity, a medical condition where so much body fat has been gained that a threat is posed to the individual's health. It gives a number which represents the weight in terms of body surface in square metres (kg/m2) by taking measurements of height and body weight.

You can be fit and healthy but still have a BMI that suggests you are overweight if you are heavily built. BMI does not take into account differences in build, and must only be used as a guide. Even if they have very little body fat, the BMI classes most male rugby players as overweight because of their larger build. For more information about weight and related subjects see Weight Loss – The Essential Guide (Need2Know). You may be eating too much of the wrong types of food if you're overweight.

Drinking

Some research published in April 2011 in the British Medical Journal showed that one in 10 cancers in men and one in 33 in women in Europe are caused by alcohol. Your risk of colorectal cancer appears to be increased by drinking large amount of alcohol – i.e. more than the weekly allowance of 14 units. Even those who were previously drinkers have a higher risk, as do those who drink below the recommended weekly limits.

Your genetic makeup

Every cell in our body contains a blueprint of our genetic material and all of this information is contained within a molecule known as DNA (deoxyribonucleic acid). DNA is composed of smaller molecules called bases and strings of these different bases are called genes and are responsible for the production of different types of proteins and other substances that our cells need to function normally. The study of inherited characteristics is called genetics. The cells lining the bowel and our skin cells are continually replacing dead cells or cells that are lost from the body, because our body's cells are constantly dividing. The DNA a cell contains is copied resulting in two identical cells with the same genetic material every single time a cell divides.

For a number of reasons, genetics is important to bowel cancer and many other cancers.

- Every time a cell divides the DNA inside it is copied. Mistakes in this copying process (mutations) do happen and this can result in a faulty gene that produces a faulty protein or other substance which does not behave as it should.

- Because mistakes are made during the copying of DNA when cells divide, there are natural processes that are designed to recognise these mistakes and correct them. Tumour suppressor genes can stop mutated cells from dividing and replicating, while other genes can make DNA repair proteins responsible for repairing the damage caused by mistakes in DNA copying. Normally, the rate at which mutations happen during the DNA copying process is controlled by the genes that produce repair proteins.

- The lining of the bowel is made of cells that divide rapidly – more rapidly than many of the body's other types of cell.

- Bowel cancer is linked to some of the genes that make up our DNA (called tumour promoter genes or oncogenes), and in people who have the disease these can be mutated or overactive. Oncogenes are involved in some way with cell division or replication. One example of an oncogene is the APC protein, which leads to an increased risk of bowel cancer in Ashkenazi Jewish people as a result of a mutated I1307K gene.

- Effectively committing suicide, some abnormal cells are controlled by a "self-destruct" mechanism known as apoptosis. A complex system of proteins and genes control this mechanism.

Our bodies ensure that all the cells they produce are normal and function appropriately through natural controls. However, in cancer cells those natural control mechanisms are not working properly and they can begin to divide uncontrollably. Researchers are now using their knowledge of the genetics of bowel cancer to increase their level of understanding on how the cancer develops and to create better treatments that are able to target cancer cells and not healthy cells. Try thinking of it like a seesaw, with oncogenes one one side and tumour suppressor genes on the other.

Our bodies ensure that all the cells they produce are normal and function appropriately through natural controls.

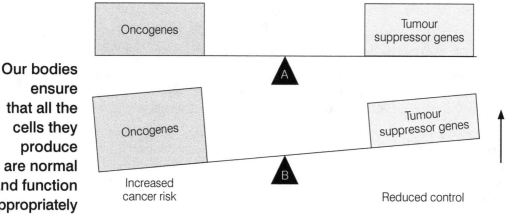

The seesaw is normally level (A) as each process balances the other. If the oncogenes become overactive (number of faulty proteins produced through mutation increases) or a mutation occurs in the gene for the DNA repair proteins (repair process is damaged), the possibility of cells becoming cancerous is increased as the normal control of rapidly dividing cells is affected (B).

This should give you some insight into understanding the importance of genetics and cancer, though in reality the science of genetics is far more complicated than the seesaw concept outlined above.

Cancer

When the normal process of replacement of cells in the body becomes uncontrolled, this can cause cancer. A growth known as a tumour forms when the cells continue to divide. These benign tumours can cause problems if their size causes them to press on surrounding tissues, for example in the brain. Cancer is considered to be a tumour whose cells spread to other parts of the body, so not all tumours are necessarily cancerous.

Cancers are described by the location of the malignant tumour (the primary site), for example bowel cancer, lung cancer, breast cancer, skin cancer and many others. Usually in the blood or the lymphatic system, cells can spread from a cancerous or malignant tumour to other parts of the body.

Metastases, or secondary tumours, are tumours that form in other parts of the body from cells that spread from the primary tumour. We'll talk about this in greater detail later on.

How does bowel cancer develop?

Several layers of tissue make up the walls of the bowel. Most cancers start as a small growth called a polyp or adenoma on the inner bowel wall. It is thought that bowel cancer develops over 5-10 years, beginning on the inner wall. The growth can spread to other layers of the bowel if left untreated and undiagnosed, and can eventually spread to other parts of the body like the prostate, bladder or womb.

In addition, bowel cancer cells can travel through the bloodstream to other more distant parts of the body and form cancers in other sites. This process is known as metastatic spread. Blood from the bowel goes directly to the liver, making this organ a common site for the development of metastatic cancer.

The lymphatic system carries fluid to and from our body tissues and is also part of the body's immune system. Vessels and swellings called lymph nodes make up the lymphatic system. One of the first places that bowel cancer can spread to is the abdomen, which has plentiful lymph nodes which can then allow the disease to spread throughout the body.

Causes of bowel cancer

Research around the world has identified a number of risk factors for bowel cancer, but we don't yet know exactly why cells lose control of their division and become cancerous. You should also remember that if you have cancer you may not necessarily have any or all of these risk factors. These risk factors do increase the likelihood of getting bowel cancer, but it's important to remember that they don't necessarily *cause* the disease.

Is this a common disease?

There are around 41,700 new bowel cancer cases in the UK every year, that's more than 110 every day (2013-2015). However, the rate at which new cases occur (incidence) has remained stable over the last ten years, so bowel cancer does not appear to be on the increase. Bowel cancer is the fourth most common cancer in the UK. It's the third most common cancer for women in the UK, with around 18,700 new cases each year. It's the third most common cancer in men after prostate and lung cancer. Patients are aged 60 and over in around 80% of cases. Throughout the world, incidence rates of bowel cancer seem to vary. The highest rates are in Europe, North America and Australasia. Western, Northern and Middle African countries and South Central Asia have the lowest incidence rates.

Bowel Cancer: Likely Outcomes

Generally survival rates over time (usually five or ten years) from diagnosis are used to express the outcomes for cancers. Overall, approximately 59% of people diagnosed with cancer will survive at least five years from diagnosis. Factors like age and how early the diagnosis is made can have an impact on the five-year survival rate. Younger patients generally have a better prognosis (outcome) than older people, while patients diagnosed at the earliest possible stage are believed to have a five year survival rate of over 95%.

In 2016, there were around 16,384 deaths from bowel cancer in the UK. Since the early 1990s, the death rate has been falling continuously – bowel cancer mortality rates decreased by 14% over the last decade (between 2004-2006 and 2014-2016). The mortality rates are likely to continue to fall, thanks to earlier diagnosis and improved treatments.

What Have We Learned?

- When we talk about bowel cancer, this usually means the large bowel (colon and rectum).

- "Cancer" is an incredibly frightening word which can prompt intense reactions and feelings. That said, our treatments are more effective than ever as our knowledge of cancer is always improving. The outlook for people with cancer is better now than ever before.

- Bowel cancer appears to have a genetic link. We don't know exactly why many people get bowel cancer, but there are some risk factors that have been identified that can increase the risk of getting the disease.

- If you're well informed about bowel cancer, you can better help your family, your friends or yourself.

- The outlook is especially good for people who are diagnosed early, but outcomes for anyone with bowel cancer are improving all the time.

Symptoms of Bowel Cancer

Symptoms to Watch Out For

nflammatory bowel disease and haemorrhoids share many of their symptoms with bowel cancer. Where the cancer located can also alter the types of symptoms the bowel cancer could cause. If the level of blood loss is high you may develop a condition known as anaemia, where the number of red blood cells in your body that carry blood to your tissues decreases, leaving you feeling very tired and breathless. Bowel cancer symptoms may include:

- Weight loss.

- Tenesmus (a straining sensation in the rectum, sometimes painful, that feels like wanting to go to the toilet but you are unable to pass any stools).

- A prolonged change in your regular bowel habits (for example diarrhoea or the stools becoming noticeably softer).

- Blood in stools or bleeding from the rectum (this can appear black or dark brown if the tumour is located towards the beginning of the bowel, or bright red if the tumour is in the rectum). Haemorrhoids can also cause spots of bright red blood on the toilet paper.

- Rectal and abdominal pains (this is the main symptom of cancer of the ascending colon).

- Doctor is able to feel a lump in your lower abdomen.

- Blood loss from your bowels can cause you to feel constantly short of breath or exhausted.

Feelings of being bloated or sick, constipation and prolonged pain in the abdomen may suggest a tumour is causing an obstruction in the bowel.

Is it Time to See a Doctor?

Talking about bowel problems or going to the toilet can be intensely embarrassing and therefore we prefer to keep bowel problems to ourselves. Inflammatory bowel diseases such as ulcerative colitis and Crohn's disease share a number of symptoms with bowel cancer, as do other conditions like piles (or haemorrhoids) which cause bleeding from the rectum. Most people find that they have a temporary condition or an illness that can be managed and that is less serious than cancer.

Some people with bowel cancer will not have any symptoms, while others will have symptoms that aren't obvious. You must see your GP urgently, however, if you experience any lasting changes to your bowel movements (like softer stools lasting for a week or more, or prolonged diarrhoea) or any persistent pain in your abdomen. Your treatment and outcome will be better the earlier bowel cancer is diagnosed, and if you get the all clear you won't have wasted your GP's time.

When to See a Specialist

Guidelines from NICE

The National Institute for Health and Clinical Excellence (NICE) is a government body of experts that issues guidance on how specific diseases should be diagnosed and managed by the NHS. It can be difficult for your GP to decide whether to refer you to a specialist, because the symptoms of bowel cancer are shared by a number of less serious conditions.

Your GP might ask you to wait and see if your symptoms improve over time in some cases, or if an infection is suspected they may prescribe antibiotics. To help GPs decide which patients to refer to a specialist, NICE have issued guidelines on the treatment of bowel cancer. Within two weeks of visiting their family doctor, according to the guidelines, people with symptoms listed in the guidelines should be referred to a specialist. This is known as an urgent referral.

The urgent referral

The guidance states that unexplained anaemia could be due to bleeding from a bowel cancer and advises GPs to refer people with unexplained anaemia for tests. In the following cases, the NICE guidelines say you should be seen by a specialist within two weeks of visiting your GP.

- Aged 40 to 59 years and have bleeding from the rectum with either a change of bowel habit towards looser stools or more frequent stools for six weeks or longer.

- Changes in bowel habit to looser or more frequent stools continuing for six or more weeks, or bleeding from the rectum for six or more weeks, where the patient is aged 60 years and older.

- A lump in the abdomen in the area of the colon or rectum (large bowel), at any age.

According to the guidelines, people are very unlikely to have cancer if they have the following symptoms but no lump in the abdomen.

- A change in normal bowel habits to harder, less frequent stools.

- Itching, pain and soreness, along with bleeding from the rectum.

- Abdominal pains with no sign that the bowel is blocked.

Within two weeks of visiting their family doctor, according to the guidelines, people with symptoms listed in the guidelines should be referred to a specialist.

What Have We Learned?

- Don't be embarrassed to see a doctor – they will deal with these problems on a daily basis and it could save your life.

- Early diagnosis of bowel cancer is critical to ensure the best possible outcome.

- Other less serious conditions share their symptoms with those of bowel cancer, which can be very vague.

- If you experience anything out of the ordinary – such as a prolonged pain or lasting change to your bowel habits – you should see your GP urgently.

- Your GP will refer you to a specialist if you are considered to be at risk.

Bowel Cancer – A Survivor's Story

Author's Introduction

have a heart condition that has (so far) been successfully treated with surgery, so in a sense I have had a life-changing event because of a medical condition and there are some similarities with living with cancer: I have to cope with life every day with the knowledge that my condition might return at any time. I cannot really appreciate what it feels like to have bowel cancer and to live with it, as I'm writing this book without having had the disease myself.

I know of two people who have had bowel cancer and one of them, Mr B, very kindly offered to speak to me about his bowel cancer to add a patient perspective to this book. Everyone knows someone who has been affected by cancer at some point in their lives. Mr B's help has been essential to the writing of this book. You can find his story below.

Mr B: My Story

Everyone knows someone who has been affected by cancer at some point in their lives. Mr B's help has been essential to the writing of this book.

I knew about bowel cancer because my mother had died from it. She was diagnosed when she was 94, and the the doctors could do very little for her at the time because the cancer was so advanced.

I have very clear memories from when I found out I had bowel cancer. It was January 2007, and I was preparing for the arrival of our first grandchild by decorating my eldest son's nursery. I was unable to finish the job, as I came down with what I thought was a flu: I was tired, had hot sweats and shivers and could not eat.

I had recently been diagnosed with Type 2 diabetes, so when I lost a lot of weight in a short time I put it down to a change in diet. I still hadn't recovered at all after ten days. One morning, I woke up to find a large, soft lump around the size of a tennis ball just above my waistline on the right side of my abdomen. It hadn't been there the night before, so I was worried.

My wife rang the emergency doctor, and we were told to go to Accident and Emergencies at the local hospital. I was admitted, and a series of X-rays and scans were carried out. In the end, a surgeon had to carry out an exploratory operation to look inside my abdomen, as the doctors weren't sure what the problem was. After the operation, I was told that my colon had split and an abscess had formed from the fluid that leaked out – this was the lump I'd found.

The surgeon explained that he'd removed part of the colon which contained a large tumour – the cause of the split – as well as the majority of the abscess. Part of the abscess has become stuck to the inner wall of my abdomen, though, so it couldn't be removed. I didn't have to have a stoma, as the surgeon had managed to sew the two ends of the colon straight back together.

The abscess and tumour were sent for analysis, and the results came back the day before I was due to be discharged. The colorectal nurse explained that the tumour had been cancer, but that it was okay because the tumour had already been removed. I was referred to the cancer team and given an MRI scan, after which the cancer specialist told me that he couldn't find any evidence of cancer. However, because the colon had split and they'd been unable to remove all of the abscess that had formed, he couldn't be sure that there were no remaining cancer cells. My choices were a combination of radiotherapy and chemotherapy, or to walk away with no further treatment.

I remembered that I'd been decorating my first grandchild's nursery when I'd fallen ill. Even though I felt guilty and upset that I hadn't been able to finish the job, I accepted the treatment because I didn't want to risk not being around to see my grandchild.

Starting in April 2007, I had 25 sessions of radiotherapy at one session per day while taking tablets of a chemotherapy drug called capecitabine. My wife and family had to take me to the hospital for treatment because the radiotherapy made me too tired to drive, but I seemed to handle the chemotherapy tablets fine to begin with. I'd been told that I might lose my hair, but that didn't happen.

The one issue with the tablets was that they caused my hands and feet to swell painfully. At one point, I wasn't able to stand up because the pain was so bad. My feet felt like they were burning, and the pain was so bad that I had to sleep with them outside the bedclothes. A week and a half before I was due to finish the course, I had to stop taking the tablets because I couldn't tolerate the pain any longer.

During the chemotherapy, I was told that I was to avoid infections at all cost as this would delay the treatment by a month. I had always been active, enjoying walking, golf, cycling and gardening, so it was frustrating that I couldn't do these things any more. I wouldn't have been able to enjoy my pastimes, even without the swelling and pain in my hands and feet.

Despite my best efforts, I developed a bowel infection the day after I finished my course of radiotherapy. I had to go back into hospital for antibiotics, as I was having bouts of severe diarrhoea every 30 minutes or so, day and night. Luckily, the infection cleared up within a few days and didn't delay my next cycle of chemotherapy.

Chemotherapy was hugely frustrating at times, as the symptoms and risk of infection kept me virtually housebound for nine months. I spent most of my time at home doing jigsaws. While I'd been told that I could exercise in moderation, I didn't feel up to it. I had to go out in the car and stay in the car when we did go out.

I felt very frustrated and depressed, but I focussed on being there for the birth of my grandchild. I needed to make sure that I was clear of cancer.

I had a number of follow-up visits with the hospital's cancer team and though nobody ever said I was cured, I was told that there was no evidence of cancer. When my grandson was born it was hugely emotional and it made the pain, anger and frustration I'd experienced during radiotherapy and chemotherapy worthwhile.

I've had two more grandchildren since that time, and I'd happily go through it all again if it meant I'd get to watch them grow up. Right now, I'm having follow-up appointments each year. Next year, I'll be able to stop meeting with the specialists as it will have been five years since my diagnosis and I'm still clear of cancer.

When I look back, I feel very lucky that my cancer was effectively removed before it was even diagnosed. I used to feel like a fraud at times, because a lot of people with bowel cancer were far more sick than me. I felt like I should have been coping better with the treatment I was receiving. I had no pain or blood loss and my bowel movements were normal. Apart from the sudden weight loss, I'd had none of the symptoms normally associated with the disease, so I didn't know how long I'd be able to live with it.

I probably wouldn't have been so accepting of my condition if I'd been diagnosed sooner, by my GP for instance. In a way I didn't feel like I had cancer because by the time I found out I had a tumour in my colon, it had already been removed.

I'm now 72 years old, and I'm living my life to the full. I haven't been on a bike since I had my operation, but I definitely want to do it again even if I can't go as far as I used to. I've always loved cycling. I go walking often and spend plenty of time in the garden, but I always want to do more because I'm enjoying life so much now. Cancer really forced me to change my perspective on life.

My digestive system has got slower since my operation and sometimes food and gas gan get trapped, so I have to keep an eye on what I eat. I have to avoid certain foods like mushrooms, tomatoes and anything overly acidic. I have to take smaller meals and have my main meal at lunchtime. These are really small prices to pay for getting my life back.

If I were to talk to someone with bowel cancer, the first thing I'd say is that it's not a killer and can be treated – sometimes even cured. The treatment can be really hard and long, though! Always make sure you have a focus in life, like your family, something you like doing or something you want to achieve. I believe that your state of mind has a big impact on how you cope with cancer. You must never give up. If you do, you'll sink into a dark abyss from which you may never escape.

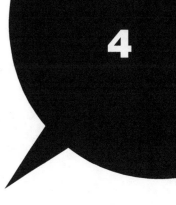

4

How Can I Avoid Bowel Cancer?

There are a number of ways to reduce the potential impact of some of the risk factors discussed previously and minimise your risk of getting bowel cancer – after all, prevention is better than a cure.

Modifying Risk Factors

We introduced the idea of modifiable and non-modifiable risk factors in the previous chapter. We'll look at ways of reducing your risk of getting the disease in this section, by examining the modifiable risk factors for bowel cancer.

Lifestyle

Smoking

For many, smoking is an addiction that seems impossible to break however there are numerous NHS Stop Smoking services available locally that can provide you with continued support and treatment to help you quit, or at the very least, to cut down. As with alcohol, ex-smokers have a higher risk compared with people who have never smoked.

Apart from all the other health-related issues associated with smoking, there's also a clear link between smoking and increased likelihood of getting bowel cancer. According to some research, most heavy smokers want to quit but are unable to do so, and giving up smoking carries some of the highest possible benefits when it comes to improving your health.

Drinking

Even small amounts of alcohol that remain below the recommended daily number of units are associated with a higher risk of bowel cancer – we discussed this in 1. The message here is to enjoy alcohol sensibly, in moderation and to have a healthy diet. Ex-drinkers also have a higher risk.

Physical activity

Walking, jogging, cycling and swimming are all exercises which are effective in giving your whole body a workout. The recommended level activity for adults is for 30 minutes of moderate exercise (such as walking) at least five days a week. The government recognises that modern lifestyles are different in that fewer people take regular exercise and this coincides with an increase in obesity in the general population.

Higher risks of bowel cancer are associated with those who don't exercise. As with all lifestyle changes, gradual changes are best, so as far as exercising is concerned, it is best to start gradually and work up, especially for those who do not exercise at all. All sorts of benefits like longer life, reducing the risk of developing diseases like diabetes, cardiovascular disease and cancer, keeping the body in good condition and feeling better can come with regular physical activity.

Especially if you are trying to change your lifestyle on your own, lifestyle changes can be incredibly difficult to make. Your chances of success will be increased if you find motivation and guidance from family and friends who are willing to work with you and change your lifestyles together.

Check the Help List for information: you can find some great guidance and information about local activities in your area through the NHS Change4Life website.

You are what you eat

Meat

The Department of Health recommends that if you currently eat more than 90g of red meat in one day you should try to cut this down to the UK average of 70g a day. As an alternative to red meat, try to include more white meat such as chicken and turkey, and more fish in your diet. One of the key findings of the EPIC study is that eating fish probably reduces the risk of developing bowel cancer, though this has not been proven for definite.

The risk of bowel cancer has been shown to be increased by red meat, and especially processed red meat. Consuming red meat in moderation is sensible – this information doesn't mean you have to stop eating it entirely, but just put more thought into the amounts you consume. For example, the recommended amount is equal to roughly three slices of ham or two standard beef burgers. White meats and fish contain less fat than red meat and are very high in protein.

GDA: Guideline Daily Amount

Many foods are now labelled with information on nutritional value and the proportion of the GDA amount that the food contains. A series of GDAs that provide guidance on how many nutrients and calories people should consume each day in order to have a healthy, balanced diet was released by the Food and Drink Federation. The GDA values are based on those for a physically active person of healthy weight, but they are guides, not targets.

GDAs for protein, sugars, saturates (saturated fat), salt, fibre, fat, carbohydrate and calories are summarised in the table overleaf.

Many foods are now labelled with information on nutritional value and the proportion of the GDA amount that the food contains.

Typical Values	Children (5-10 years)	Women	Men
Calories	1,800 kcal	2,000 kcal	2,500 kcal
Carbohydrate	220g	230g	300g
Fat	70g	70g	95g
Fibre	15g	24g	24g
Protein	24g	45g	55g
Salt	4g	6g	6g
Saturates	20g	20g	30g
Sugars	85g	90g	120g

Although it's recommended not to exceed the GDA for calories, sugars, fat, saturates and salt, people of certain weights, ages, activity levels or genders may need to eat amounts that are larger or smaller than the GDA.

The purpose of this information is to help you make informed decisions about what foods you eat in order to have a more balanced, nutritious diet.

Roughage

Fibre (also previously known as roughage) comes from plant-based foods and cannot be digested by the human body. Fibre can be either soluble or insoluble. If you want to keep your bowels healthy and fully functional, it's essential that your diet contains fibre. Fibre reduces the likelihood of bowel cancer as it speeds up the removal of toxins and waste, stopping them from spending too much time in contact with the bowel.

Soluble fibre is found in fruit and vegetables with apples, strawberries and legumes being rich sources. Stools are made softer and easier to pass by soluble fibre, which absorbs the water in the bowel. It can also help to control blood sugar levels and reduce cholesterol.

Insoluble fibre makes the stools soft and bulky and quicker and easier to pass out of the body, preventing constipation. The human body is completely unable to digest insoluble fibre as it consists primarily of a substance called cellulose.

The recommended guideline daily amount for fibre intake for adults per day is 18g, although according to the British Nutrition Foundation the average daily fibre intake in the UK is 12g, meaning that most of us do not have enough fibre in our current diets. The table below summarises the different sources of soluble and insoluble fibre. Both insoluble and soluble fibre can be found in some foods, such as beans and oats.

Insoluble Fibre	Beans
	Brown rice
	Lentils
	Nuts
	Oats
	Okra
	Seeds
	Skins of fruit
	Wheat bran
	Wholemeal bread, cereals and pasta
	Whole-wheat bread
Soluble Fibre	Barley
	Citrus fruit (oranges, lemons, limes)
	Legumes (peas, beans, lentils, peanuts)
	Oats/Oat bran
	Pears
	Potatoes
	Purple passion fruit
	Some beans (black beans, navy beans, kidney beans)
	Soy

How much fibre is in my food?

The next table shows a summary of popular foods and the average amount of fibre they contain. It's useful to have an idea of how much fibre commonly eaten foods contain if you want to increase the amount in your diet. There has to be 6g of fibre per 100g weight or 100ml volume for a food to be classed as "high fibre". There has to be at least 3g of fibre per 100g weight or 100ml volume for it to be labelled "source of fibre".

Food	How much?	Grammes of Fibre
Almonds	13g	1.3
Apple	100g	2.4
Baked beans	150g	6.8
Baked potato (with skin)	Whole potato	5
Banana	100g	1.5
Cereal (e.g. Bran Flakes, Fruit & Fibre)	One bowl (30g)	4-7
Lentils	One portion (80g)	1.5
Pasta (wholewheat)	One portion (90g)	9
Strawberries	100g	1.5
White bread	One slice	0.8
Wholemeal bread	One slice	3-4

The key findings of the EPIC study have shown that a high fibre diet reduces the risk of bowel cancer.

The key findings of the EPIC study have shown that a high fibre diet reduces the risk of bowel cancer. In addition, it seems that there are also additional gains from a high fibre diet. An increase of no more than 5g in a week is probably a good idea. It's essential that you have fibre in your diet, but it's still possible to take too much fibre – too much can cause you to become deficient in minerals like calcium, zinc and iron.

In order to avoid these problems, it's best to build up the amount of fibre you consume gradually. Note the massive difference between the fibre contents of wholemeal bread and white. Simply switching from white to wholemeal bread can make a big impact on your daily fibre intake, as it contains around 4-5 times as much fibre as white bread. It appears that fibre helps to stop polyps from transforming into cancer, and from developing in the first place. A 2013 study in the British Medical Journal also concluded that "Greater dietary fibre intake is associated with a lower risk of both cardiovascular disease and coronary heart disease. Findings are aligned with general recommendations to increase fibre intake."[1] So it seems that a diet that's high in fibre does much more than just reducing the risk of bowel cancer!

---

1   https://www.ncbi.nlm.nih.gov/pubmed/24355537

Watching your weight

Maintaining a healthy weight will reduce your risk if you are overweight or obese. Losing weight is a lifestyle change and requires dedication and perseverance but the health benefits are substantial. Support from your family and friends is invaluable, as are organisations such as Weight Loss Resources (www.weightlossresources.co.uk) and WeightWatchers (www.weightwatchers.co.uk), where you can join others who all have the same goal in mind. There's a strong link between obesity and an increased risk of bowel cancer, as we've already discussed. A good guide to your healthy weight range is the BMI, and you should aim to have yours no higher than 25. A healthy balanced diet combined with regular exercise is the best way to lose weight.

Screenings

In the UK there are a number of different screening programmes in place for bowel cancer. Healthy people who exhibit no symptoms may be screened for bowel cancer to look for early signs of the disease. You will normally be informed of the results within a fortnight. Since the risk of bowel cancer increases with age, all people aged 60-69 are sent a stool testing kit to test for blood (faecal occult blood or FOB test) every two years.

The FOB test is simple to use. The proportion of abnormal results (positive FOB tests) is small (only about 2%) and the presence of blood in the stools does not necessarily imply that the cause is cancer. People with an abnormal result will be invited to attend a bowel screening centre, where a more detailed examination will be carried out and a colonoscopy may be offered. Colonoscopy is carried out at a hospital as a day case (meaning that you can go home on the same day after having the test). This procedure checks for abnormalities by passing a small flexible tube with a camera and light (endoscope) into the rectum and up into the colon.

Nationwide coverage has now been achieved by the BCSP (bowel cancer screening programme), which started in England in 2006 by the NHS (National Health Service). People in Wales are given FOB tests every two years from age 60-69 and in Scotland every two years from age 50-74. The screening kit can be requested by people over the age of 70 by contacting the NHS BCSP. Tests are offered every two years to people aged 60-69 in Northern Ireland as part of a screening programme that was started in April 2010. Stool samples are wiped on test cards, before being sealed and sent for analysis in a laboratory. The NHS bowel cancer screening programme website (included in the

Help List at the end of this book) has full information on how to use the FOB test kit. Be aware of the symptoms of bowel cancer and see your GP if you are at all worried, as a negative FOB test doesn't necessarily rule out cancer.

Colonoscopies are used to examine the full length of the colon and allow the doctor as the endoscope passes along to look at the lining of the colon on a monitor. Just before you have the colonoscopy you will be given a sedative (a drug designed to relax you) and the procedure normally lasts between 30 minutes and an hour. The bowel needs to be completely clear of faeces, so you'll be asked to follow a special diet and drink plenty of water in the days before the test, as well as being given laxatives.

A second FOB test will be requested for about 20 out of every 1,000 people. Of these, 16 are likely to be given a colonoscopy, around two will have cancer, six will have polyps and eight will have no notable abnormalities.

A clinical trial in the UK using an endoscope to examine the sigmoid colon, the lower part of the large bowel (flexible sigmoidoscopy) and the surgical removal of any polyps found showed that this could prevent the development of bowel cancer, as the disease usually develops slowly from polyps. Flexible sigmoidoscopy is a similar procedure to the colonoscopy outlined above, but it is quicker (usually no more than about 25 minutes) as only the lower part of the large bowel (sigmoid colon and rectum) are examined.

The results of this clinical trial showed that, in those people who had the sigmoidoscopy screen, the incidence of colorectal cancer was reduced by 33% and mortality (deaths) by 43%. For 11 years, this large study followed 170,000 patients, just over 40,000 of whom were given a single flexible sigmoidoscopy. Flexible sigmoidoscopy screenings offered once to people aged between 55 and 64 offers long-lasting protection from colorectal cancer and is highly beneficial, according to the study's findings. You will be given an enema before the procedure to flush any faeces from the sigmoid colon and rectum. Colonoscopy and flexible sigmoidoscopy are prepared for in similar ways. If the GI tract needs to be completely clear, you may be asked to follow a special diet in the days leading up to the test.

Medicines

Daily doses of aspirin (75-300mg) were found in a recent clinical study to reduce the risk of dying from bowel cancer by 35%, and to reduce the incidence of bowel cancer by 24% over 20 years. More than 14,000 patients with bowel cancer were involved in the study. With the benefits of colonoscopy and sigmoidoscopy to screen for bowel cancer, there is an appropriate time to discuss starting on aspirin. The decision as to whether aspirin would be of benefit would depend on a doctor's opinion and the risk the individual has of developing bowel cancer (i.e. if they have FAP, ulcerative colitis or Crohn's disease), as long-term use of aspirin can increase the risk of bleeding in the bowel and stomach ulcers. Without at least discussing it with your doctor, it's not advisable to take any form of preventative medicine if you have no obvious risk of bowel cancer and are otherwise healthy.

What Have We Learned?

- Early diagnosis of bowel cancer through screening has been proven to save lives. It's really important that you attend if you're invited to a screening for bowel cancer.

- To reduce your risk of getting the disease, there are a number of risk factors that you can modify:

- Enjoy alcohol in moderation and if you are a smoker then try to quit or at least cut down.

- Stick to the guideline daily amounts for calories, protein, carbohydrate, sugars, fat, saturates, fibre and salt.

- Try to include plenty of fibre (at least 18g per day) in your diet.

- Consume a balanced, nutritious diet with plenty of lean protein (like fish and white meat), fresh fruit and vegetables. Each day, try not to eat more than 70g of red meat.

- Try to maintain a healthy weight for your height by getting plenty of exercise.

- A doctor may recommend a medical treatment such as aspirin if you're at a higher risk of bowel cancer.

5

Treating Bowel Cancer

nce the cancer has been staged (see Five!) the doctor can then plan the best course for treatment. What stage a cancer is at (how advanced it is) will determine how it's treated. Surgery, radiotherapy and chemotherapy are the three main options for treating bowel cancer. These treatments can also be given in combination with each other, for example radiotherapy is often given at the same time as chemotherapy and is known as chemoradiotherapy or chemoradiation. The techniques can be carried out individually or one after the other – for example, chemotherapy may be used after surgery to stop cancer cells spreading to other parts of the body or reduce the likelihood of the cancer recurring. Cancer cells can be treated more effectively by combining different treatments.

Chemotherapy

There are a wide variety of anticancer drugs and they work in different ways. The use of drugs to treat cancer is known as chemotherapy. Most chemotherapy drugs work systemically (throughout the entire body) and they do not attack just the cancer cells but healthy cells as well.

Different drugs will have different modes of action, and in most cases they will be given in combination. The likelihood of response is improved in this way. Because they affect all dividing cells, all anticancer drugs have a number of side effects.

Nausea and vomiting

The most commonly used drug for bowel cancer, 5-FU, causes a moderate amount of nausea and this can usually be easily controlled with anti-emetics. Vomiting (being sick) and nausea (feeling sick) are caused by all chemotherapy drugs to a certain extent. At the time you start your chemotherapy it's common practice to five you an antiemetic – a drug to stop you being sick – for this reason.

Chemotherapy side effects

It is important to remember that side effects of chemotherapy are temporary and will disappear after chemotherapy is finished. Side effects will be most noticeable in the hair, skin and cells lining the GI tract and bone marrow because these are the cells that divide the most rapidly, and are the non-cancer cells that chemotherapy will affect the most.

Diarrhoea

One risk of prolonged or severe diarrhoea is dehydration (fluid loss) as the water is not being absorbed from your food, and in these cases you can be given treatments to help stop the diarrhoea and replace lost fluids. Chemotherapy drugs often cause this problem. The treatment can damage healthy cells in the bowel, leading to diarrhoea. The stools become very watery because cells are no longer able to absorb nutrients and water from the food as they should.

Mouth ulcers

Inflammation and soreness of the lining of the mouth, sometimes along with ulcers, is caused by mucositis. If it's a real problem you may be given antiseptic mouthwashes for any infected ulcers, as well as painkillers, as it can be difficult to eat, drink or swallow with this condition.

Suppression of the bone marrow

The red blood cells (those that bring oxygen to our tissues through veins and arteries), white cells (those that fight infection and make up our immune system) and platelets (those that allow blood clots to form when we're injured) are produced in the bone marrow, which makes up the central part of may of our bones such as the hip bone, sternum (breastbone) and leg bones. Chemotherapy drugs often affect the bone marrow, which is highly active and constantly releasing red cells, white cells and platelets into our bloodstreams. This can result in a reduced ability to fight infections as white cell numbers drop, problems with blood not clotting properly after injury or spontaneous bleeding (nosebleeds are common) as platelet counts drop, or anaemia and tiredness as the number of red cells being produced by the bone marrow falls. A process called bone marrow suppression occurs when chemotherapy kills many of the bone marrow cells, reducing the amount of cells the marrow can produce.

Most people have lowered levels of white cells during chemotherapy, but if the counts are very low then there are drugs that can boost white cell production or transfusions of white cells can be given. You may be given antibiotics as treatment if you are suffering from infections. Anaemia as a result of a low red cell count can be treated with blood boosting drugs or a blood transfusion if necessary, while platelet transfusions can help restore the platelet counts towards normal if bleeding problems become serious.

You may be given antibiotics as treatment if you are suffering from infections.

Alopecia – hair loss

Hair loss or thinning is commonly experienced by those having chemotherapy. This can be especially devastating for some. However, as with most of the side effects of chemotherapy, hair will almost always grow back after chemotherapy has finished. While some people may lose very little hair, others will lose most if not all of their hair. The type of chemotherapy drugs being used as well as differences from person to person will determine the amount of hair that is lost. Those that do lose a lot of hair tend to lose it in clumps as the treatment progresses. Counselling, advice, temporary hair pieces and wigs and other forms of specialist help and support are available through the NHS.

Receiving Your Chemotherapy

The treatment will be given by specially trained cancer doctors (oncologists) and/ or nurses. Many hospitals have specialist chemotherapy units, where your treatment will need to be started as the drugs used in chemotherapy are very powerful. In most cases you will be asked to remain in the chemotherapy unit while you are having the treatment, allowing the doctors and nurses to make sure that everything is happening as it should. Once started, some treatments can be given at home and in this case a doctor or nurse will visit to give the treatment. A large vein inside your chest can be used (sometimes referred to as a central line), though most chemotherapy drugs are delivered through needles into the blood vessels in your arm. You may be allowed to go home earlier if you're treated using drugs like capecitabine, which is given as a capsule or pill, or if you receive your chemotherapy drugs in the form of a rapid injection (bolus).

Your treatment will most likely consist of a series of cycles – often with a rest between each cycle to allow the body to recover before the next cycle starts – as chemotherapy drugs are given as a treatment course. Courses of chemotherapy are usually 4-6 cycles long, although they may be longer than this, so you will need to go to the hospital regularly to have your treatment. For instance, a common treatment cycle will be 28 days long with a seven-day rest period.

Surgical Treatment

With very small tumours surgery alone may be sufficient followed by regular follow-up visits to make sure that the cancer has gone. Any treatment that is given after the primary treatment (in this case surgery) is known as adjuvant treatment. About 80% of bowel tumours can be removed using surgery. In very advanced cancer, the tumour might be considered inoperable.

When the tumour has grown beyond a certain size, surgery may still be possible but would involve the removal of a significant part of the bowel which would interfere with the normal function of the bowel and requires a stoma (we'll talk about this later in the book). The most effective treatment for bowel cancer is surgery, which can be really helpful if tumours haven't spread.

Surgery offers the best chance of a cure for bowel cancer if all of the tumour can be removed. The tumour – as well as the margin, an area of healthy tissue surrounding the tissue, to ensure all cancer cells are removed – is resected (removed) by a surgeon. Most bowel cancers are too large and advanced to be treated by surgery alone, unfortunately. If this is the case, further treatment such as adjuvant chemotherapy may be needed after surgery.

Serious complications such as bleeding may prevent a surgeon from removing a tumour completely if it has grown too large or spread into other parts of the body. Treatment may include chemotherapy and radiotherapy to shrink the tumour and keep it under control in these situations, though the surgeon may still be able to remove part of the tumour (this is known as debulking).

After the tumour has shrunk, it may then be possible to remove it entirely. Otherwise, radiotherapy or chemotherapy may be given before the surgery to allow the surgeon to remove all of the cancer by first shrinking the tumour. This is known as neoadjuvant treatment. In cases where a tumour is inoperable, the tumour is so large or has invaded so many other organs and tissues that the risk to the patient far outweighs the potential benefits, so surgery is not considered appropriate. In these cases, all that can be done is to give the patient the best patient the best possible care for the rest of their life by controlling the cancer, rather than trying to cure it. Not all patients with bowel cancer can be cured, though the majority can be, as it's possible for the disease to metastatise or spread to the lymph nodes.

Bowel Cancer Surgeries

Colectomy

A colectomy is surgery that removes part of the colon that is affected by cancer. In sigmoid colectomy the sigmoid colon is removed whilst removal of the entire colon is known as total colectomy. If a section of colon is removed from the right side, the procedure is known as a right hemicolectomy. The procedure is known as a left hemicolectomy if the removed section comes from the left side of the colon. A transverse colectomy is an operation that removes part of the transverse colon.

In the case of a total colectomy the lower part of the small bowel (ileum) may need to be used to create a stoma (ileostomy) and in some cases this can be permanent. Anastomosis is a procedure where the surgeon rejoins the two healthy ends of the bowel once the cancer-bearing tissue has been removed. The surgeon may fit a temporary stoma – which is an opening in the body wall that the bowel is stitched to so that food waste can be collected outside the body in a stoma bag – if the bowel needs time to heal, or else the anastomosis might be carried out straight away. The two ends of bowel will be rejoined and the temporary stoma reversed once the damaged area of the bowel has healed.

Local resection

In a procedure known as a local resection, a tumour can be removed along with a small margin of healthy tissue provided the tumour is still very small and hasn't spread beyond the bowel lining. In rectal cancer, local resection is known as transanal resection. An endoscope with a cutting tool attached is used for this procedure.

TME – total mesenteric excision

Surgery for rectal cancer may require a temporary stoma. Along with the tumour and a margin of healthy tissue, the mesentery is routinely removed in rectal cancer. Any cancer cells that spread are likely to be found in the mesentery, as it contains lymph nodes. A permanent stoma will be needed if the entire rectum needs to be removed.

Any cancer cells that spread are likely to be found in the mesentery, as it contains lymph nodes.

Bowel Cancer: Commonly Used Chemo Drugs

Folinic acid

A planned course of chemotherapy is known as a regimen. A combination of 5-FU (see below) and folinic acid (also known as leucovorin) is often given to patients, as it's more effective than 5-FU alone.

Different doses of 5-FU are given at different times of a treatment period. Various dosages of both drugs have been used over various time periods, and the combination of the two is easy to give by infusion or intravenous bolus. The de Gramont regimen is very effective in metastatic disease, combining a high dose of folinic acid with infusion and bolus doses of 5-FU. Body surface area in square metres (m2) is used to calculate the dose of may chemotherapy drugs.

A 2-hour infusion on days 1 and 2 of a two week cycle with 200mg/m2 folinic acid:

- Days 1 and 2: 400mg/m2 5-FU as i.v. (intravenous bolus).
- Days 1 and 2: 600mg/m2 5-FU as an infusion over 22 hours.

This is repeated every 2 weeks in most cases.

5-FU – 5-fluorouracil

5-FU is usually given through a large blood vessel, directly into the bloodstream, either as an injection of a single large dose (bolus) or by introducing the drug more gradually through a drip or using a pump over several hours or longer (infusion). 5-FU can be given by infusion into the hepatic portal vein (the main vein that carries blood to the liver from the bowel) for treating liver metastases. Tumours in the liver can receive a high dose of the drug using this method. A hand-foot syndrome known as palmar-plantar erythema can occur in people who are given the drug by infusion. This is not usually serious for most people and they can carry on with their treatment, though for some it can be quite frightening, causing soreness, peeling and reddening of the skin on feet and hands. The doctor can choose to delay treatment until the condition clears up if it does become a problem.

5-fluorouracil is similar to one of the components of DNA, uracil, but with a slightly different structure. For more than 25 years, this drug has been used in bowel cancer treatment.

5-FU helps to prevent the cancer cells from producing new DNA by interfering with the process where DNA is copied when they divide. The drug helps to stop cancer cells from dividing as a result. Folinic acid is often used in combination with 5-FU. Although some will develop mucositis, bone marrow suppression, diarrhoea and nausea/vomiting, most people cope well with 5-FU which is considered to be a mild treatment with few side effects.

Irinotecan

Irinotecan is a powerful drug and its side effects include nausea/vomiting, delayed onset diarrhoea which can be serious and need prompt treatment, bone marrow suppression and hair loss. Irinotecan inhibits an enzyme called topoisomerase 1, which unzips the DNA structure. DNA cannot copy itself if it's unable to unwind during cell division – a process which can be stopped by the drug irinotecan. Cancer cells cannot replicate as a result.

Other chemotherapy drugs like 5-FU and folinic acid are often used in combination with irinotecan, which is usually given through an intravenous infusion.

Eloxatin – oxaliplatin

Cancer cell division and replication can be inhibited by oxaliplatin, a drug based on the precious metal platinum which interferes with the production of DNA. Oxaliplatin is a well-tolerated platinum-based drug (many drugs in this class, especially cisplatin, are highly toxic). The response rate of the de Gramont regimen of 5-FU and folinic acid can be doubled when combined with oxaliplatin, which is very effective in the treatment of colorectal cancer.

Sensory peripheral neuropathy, a condition which affects the nerves causing tingling and numbness in the hands and feet, along with nausea and bone marrow suppression are the most common side effects of this drug. If sensory peripheral neuropathy becomes a real issue, the doctor will often reduce the dose of the drug to see if the condition improves as it is related to the dose of oxaliplatin – however, in most cases this side effect is only mild.

Tegafur

Tegafur has similar side effects to 5-FU and capecitabine as the drugs are very similar. Tegafur is a prodrug (see below) of fluorouracil, like capecitabine. When used as first-line treatment of metastatic bowel cancer, it's given as a tablet with uracil (which helps to prevent the breakdown of fluorouracil, the active part of tegafur) and folinic acid.

Xeloda – capecitabine

Capecitabine can be given with uracil and folinic acid as first-line (initial) chemotherapy treatment for metastatic bowel cancer or as adjuvant treatment (combined with oxaliplatin) following surgery in advanced (TNM stage 3 or Dukes C) bowel cancer. This drug is inactive and only converted into an active form when inside the body or inside the tumour – this type of drug is called a prodrug. It means that capecitabine is converted into its active form, fluorouracil (5-FU) when it is inside the tumour, and there is a markedly lower chance of it attacking healthy, non-cancerous cells, which helps to reduce its side effects. Targets are generally selected more carefully by prodrugs.

While most chemotherapy drugs used to treat bowel cancer have to be injected, capecitabine can be taken orally (by mouth) – another advantage.

The drugs 5-FU and capecitabine are very similar, so they have similar side effects.

Side Effects of Radiotherapy

Radiotherapy side effects are usually divided into those that appear while radiotherapy is being given (early effects) or those that may develop some time after the course of treatment has finished (late effects). Every person who is treated with radiotherapy will tolerate it differently; some may experience no side effects at all, whereas others might develop side effects that make them feel physically ill or interfere with their normal daily activities. There are side effects caused by the radiation beam passing through normal tissue to reach the tumour, even though radiotherapy is very precise in only treating the tumour tissues. The location of the tumour and whether or not any other structures and organs are affected (like the liver, kidneys or spinal cord) will also determine the treatment's side effects.

Late effects

Late effects appear many months after radiotherapy has finished and may include fibrosis (thickening and hardening) of skin or bleeding and holes (perforation) appearing in the affected bowel tissue. Exposure to radiotherapy can result in a permanent change in otherwise normal cells and tissues. This is what causes late effects, which are more serious than early effects. Most people will not experience late effects of radiotherapy as, fortunately, they are rare.

Side effects during the treatment

These can be as a result of the radiation damaging normal calls, or can be generalised – such as becoming depressed or anxious because of the constant trips to the hospital, or feeling lethargic and fatigued during treatment. Diarrhoea is a common problem as the normal function of the non-cancerous bowel is disrupted. Flaking, reddening, rashes and soreness can all occur in bowel cancer when radiotherapy damages the skin in the path of the beam.

The early effects will eventually disappear once the treatment has finished and the cells have repaired themselves, as they are a result of the interference with the function of normal cells by radiotherapy.

Radiation Therapy

If your tumour is large and difficult to remove using surgery, you may be given radiotherapy after surgery (postoperatively, adjuvant treatment) to help destroy any cancer cells left behind or if there are cancer cells in the lymph nodes. Radiotherapy is usually used to treat rectal cancer and is normally given in addition to other treatments. Modern radiotherapy machines are able to focus the beam of particles to the exact size and shape of the tumour, which limits the damage to surrounding healthy cells and the tissue that the particles have to travel through to reach the tumour.

Radiotherapy is usually given at regular intervals for about five weeks, although the time may be longer or shorter than this. Cancer cells are killed through this technique by pointing a high-intensity beam of radioactive particles directly at the tumour. External beam radiotherapy is a type of radiotherapy that's delivered to the body from the outside as a beam of particles.

The radiographer or doctor will draw a series of marks on the skin to allow the radiotherapy machine to deliver the treatment to exactly the right place. Chemotherapy drugs such as 5-FU are often given at the same time as they make cancer cells more sensitive to the effects of radiotherapy, and radiotherapy can be given preoperatively (neoadjuvant treatment, ahead of surgery) to make the tumour easier to remove by shrinking it.

The treatment is given in fractions (in other words little and often) as this seems to be most effective and patients cope better with smaller amounts of treatment given at regular intervals. Radioactive particles can be contained inside a tube and delivered inside the body using a newer internal radiotherapy treatment called brachytherapy. This is used to shrink the tumour so that it can be removed surgically – in rectal cancer, the brachytherapy tube is inserted into the rectum through the anus, placed close to the tumour and left in place for the duration of the treatment. A machine called a simulator is used to plan external beam radiotherapy. It moves in exactly the same way as the radiotherapy machine will during actual treatment, but takes X-rays instead of producing radiotherapy. How much radiotherapy to use, as well of the size and shape of the tumour, will be determined by the doctor using these X-rays (and CT scans if necessary). You can receive your radiotherapy for real once all of the planning is finished. You could be asked to have radiotherapy daily without a break, but in most cases a course of radiotherapy would involved daily treatments on weekdays with a rest period (no treatment) at the weekend.

What Have We Learned?

- The main treatment for bowel cancer is surgery and it offers the best chance of cure.

- Chemotherapy and radiotherapy affect healthy cells too and are associated with a number of side effects, those these will eventually disappear after treatment stops.

- The stage the cancer is at when it's diagnosed will determine the treatment of bowel cancer.

- To make the treatment of the disease as effective as possible, other treatments such as chemotherapy and radiotherapy can be given before (neoadjuvant), during or after surgery (adjuvant).

6

Bowel Cancer Diagnosis

As we've already discussed, it's vital that you get diagnosed early on if you want your treatment to have the best possible outcome – those cancers that are diagnosed early on can be cured with surgery, so the earlier the diagnosis the better the outcome.

Staging of Bowel Cancer

The process of staging allows the doctor to determine how large the cancer is, whether it has spread, and if so, by how much. Bowel cancer is "staged", just like most other cancers. Bowel cancer is staged using two staging systems.

TNM staging system

A wide range of cancers are staged using the tumour, node, metastases (TNM) staging system.

Tumour size and spreading are described by T, which is subdivided according to size into T1, T2, T3 and T4.

- T1: The tumour is only in the lining of the bowel.

- T2: The tumour is also in the bowel's muscle wall.

- T3: The tumour has grown into other structures and organs adjoining the bowel, or into the peritoneum (outermost layer of the bowel).

- T4: The tumour has grown beyond the peritoneum, into other areas of the bowel, or into other structures or organs adjoining the bowel.

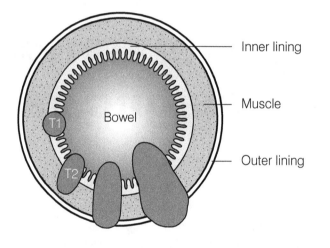

T stages of bowel cancer

Lymph node involvement is described by N, which is subdivided according to how many lymph nodes are involved (if any) into N0, N1 and N2.

- N0: Lymph nodes close to the bowel contain no cancer cells.

- N1: Cancer cells are found in 1-3 of the lymph nodes close to the bowel.

- N2: Cancer cells are found in 4+ of the lymph nodes at least 3cm from the bowel, or in the lymph nodes close to the main blood vessels around the bowel.

Metastases are described by M, which is subdivided into M0 and M1.

- M0: Other parts of the body outside of the bowel are not affected by the tumour.

- M1: Other parts of the body, such as the liver, are affected by the tumour.

The next table summarises the 5 stages of bowel cancer (0, 1, 2, 3 and 4). The T, N and M elements are combined when using the TNM system to describe the stage of cancer and will vary depending on how advanced or otherwise the cancer is. For example, a tumour that is confined to the bowel lining (T1) with no cancer cells in the lymph nodes (N0) and no spread to other parts of the body (M0) could be written as T1, N0, M0.

Stage	TNM Classification	Description
0	T0, TIS (Tumour in situ)	TIS or Stage 0 is an early stage of bowel cancer. There are cancer cells in your bowel lining, but they're completely contained. There is little risk of any cancer cells having spread.
1	T1,N0,M0 or T2,N0,M0	The tumour has grown into the lining of the bowel (T1) or has grown into the muscle wall (T2).
2a 2b	T3,N0,M0 T4,N0,M0	The cancer has grown into the outer covering of the bowel. The tumour has grown through the peritoneum and into the other areas of the bowel or other organs or structures adjoining the bowel (T4) but has not spread to the lymph nodes or other parts of the body.
3a 3b 3c	T1,N1,M0 or T2,N1,M0 T3,N1,M0 or T4,N1,M0 T(any),N2,M0	The cancer is still in the inner layer of the bowel wall, or has grown into the muscle layer. Between 1 to 3 nearby lymph nodes may contain cancer cells. The tumour has grown through the peritoneum and into other areas of the bowel or other organs or structures adjoining the bowel (T4) and between one and three close lymph nodes have cancer cells in them. The cancer can be any size. It has spread to 4 or more nearby lymph nodes. The cancer has not spread to any other part of the body.
4	T(any),N(any),M1	The cancer has spread to other parts of the body such as the liver or lungs through either the bloodstream or the lymphatic system.

The system has been designed to ensure the most accurate description of the stage of bowel cancer, even though it may seem complicated.

The system has been designed to ensure the most accurate description of the stage of bowel cancer, even though it may seem complicated. This means the doctor is able to work out the best treatment for the condition.

Dukes' staging system

This system is gradually being replaced by the TNM system. The Dukes' system has four stages: A, B, C and D. A British doctor called Cuthbert Dukes created the Dukes' staging system for classifying colorectal cancer in 1932. Subdivisions to stages B and C were added when the system was adapted in 1954. A summary of the full staging system can be found in the table below.

Dukes Stage	Description
A	The cancer is in the inner lining of the bowel, or is growing slightly into the muscle layer.
B1	The tumour has grown into the muscle wall of the bowel but not beyond it.
B2	The tumour is penetrating the muscle wall, but the lymph nodes are not involved.
C1	The tumour has grown into the muscle wall of the bowel but not beyond it. Lymph nodes are involved.
C2	The tumour is penetrating the muscle wall and lymph nodes are involved.
D	The tumour has spread to other parts of the body (metastasis).

How Is Bowel Cancer Diagnosed?

Virtual colonoscopy

Bowel cancer is diagnosed through a number of different techniques. For example, a doctor may perform a "virtual colonoscopy". Virtual colonoscopy looks at the whole of the abdomen and not just the lining of the bowel so it can be useful for showing any tumours that might have formed outside the bowel. The virtual colonoscopy technique can show the presence of polyps or other unusual or abnormal changes to the bowel and pinpoint their exact location. Computerised tomography (CT) scanning is used during this procedure. Three-dimensional images or image "slices" through the body are produced by a computer when it processes a series of X-ray images taken by the CT scanner. A small tube is placed into the rectum to pump in air to make it easier to obtain images of the large bowel.

The rectum needs to be empty of stools for the procedure, so preparation generally involves the use of laxatives and an enema. Unlike colonoscopy and sigmoidoscopy you do not need to be given a drug to make you relax (sedative). Virtual colonoscopy is a short procedure (usually about ten minutes) and has the added advantage of being more comfortable and simpler to perform than a colonoscopy or sigmoidoscopy as it doesn't require an endoscope. It's also known as CTC or computerised tomography colonography. Afterwards, you won't have to rely on another person to assist you and can simply return home to continue with your daily activities. The procedure cannot be used to take biopsies, unfortunately.

Colonoscopy and sigmoidoscopy (endoscopy)

Colonoscopy and sigmoidoscopy procedures were explained in the previous chapters. During a sigmoidoscopy or colonoscopy, a biopsy (small sample tissue) is taken from any polyps that are identified – this is bowel cancer is usually diagnosed. The presence of any cancer cells in the biopsy will be detected through analysis in a laboratory.

Ultrasound

A probe is used in this technique to send sound waves through the body. A monitor is then used to display reflected sound from organs and structures within the body as they are picked up by the probe. In order to stage any cancer found in the lining of the rectum and colon, the technique can be combined with an endoscope – this process is known as EUS (endoscopic ultrasound).

MRI scans

MRI can be used to accurately determine how far a tumour has spread within the bowel wall or to look for the presence of metastases in the liver. A machine that generates a very powerful magnetic field is used in MRI (magnetic resonance imaging), but otherwise it's a scanning procedure very similar to CT scanning. Tumours may be more easily seen through MRI than with other techniques as the images obtained are very highly detailed.

Differential diagnosis

The process of ruling out other conditions is called differential diagnosis and involves the doctor looking at the symptoms and determining which condition most closely matches these to help make a diagnosis. Before the diagnosis of cancer is made, it's important to rule out the number of conditions which share the same symptoms as those of bowel cancer.

Barium enemas

Barium is a solution that is given to coat the lining of the bowel like a paint. A barium enema requires the bowel to be completely clear of any faeces and so preparation involves strong laxatives. Normal X-rays are unable to show enough detail as the bowel contains air. However, barium allows the lining to be shown clearly in the X-ray as white areas. Those preparing for a barium enema will be asked to drink only water and not eat any food for 24 hours.

Once the biopsy samples are obtained they are sent to a laboratory where the samples are viewed under the microscope to test for the presence of cancer cells.

What Is a Biopsy?

A sample of tissue that's taken for analysis is referred to as a "biopsy". Once the biopsy samples are obtained they are sent to a laboratory where the samples are viewed under the microscope to test for the presence of cancer cells. Biopsy tissue can be taken from a lymph node, tumour or polyp for bowel cancer.

A special surgical tool contained within the endoscope is usually used to take a tumour or biopsy during a colonoscopy or sigmoidoscopy. A different technique is required to test lymph nodes, as they are located outside the bowel. Instead, needle biopsy is used – this is where a fine needle is inserted into the lymph node under local anaesthetic. This might not be enough for analysis of bowel cancer, however, as needle biopsy only provides a small amount of tissue. A sample of lymph node can be surgically removed during an open biopsy procedure instead, where a small incision is made under local anaesthetic.

The best lymph node from which to take a biopsy can be found by the doctor through a special technique called sentinal lymph node biopsy, which is often used in cancer. Here, the sentinal (first) lymph node into which the cancer cells would spread is identified by injecting a small amount of dye into the tumour. The sentinal and perhaps one or two neighbouring lymph nodes are then used for biopsy.

What Have We Learned?

- Diagnostic techniques for bowel cancer can include:

- Barium enema

- Colonoscopy and sigmoidoscopy (endoscopy)

- MRI

- Ultrasound

- A biopsy is a sample of tissue taken to be tested for the presence of cancer cells.

- It's really important you get your bowel cancer diagnosed early if you want the best possible outcome.

- To determine the best treatment approach, bowel cancer is "staged" by the doctor. Bowel cancer will be staged using one of two systems. Dukes' system is currently being phased out in favour of TNM.

7

Life with Bowel Cancer

Processing Your Diagnosis

You may feel as if your whole world has been turned inside out and that you have no control over your life anymore. We all know somebody who either has or has had cancer so public awareness of the disease is very high and it is much less of a taboo subject than it once was. Being told be a doctor that you have cancer can be devastating and distressing for the majority of people. Some people decide to keep the news to themselves so as not to shock or worry others, but unfortunately cancer does not go away and a disease like this cannot be hidden forever. There are a number of bowel cancer organisations and support group that can provide valuable support.

Talking to your friends and family about your diagnosis is very important – people are very supportive when they learn that a friend or a loved one has cancer. Feeling afraid and abandoned is very common. You should not have to deal with this on your own – cancer is a serious and potentially life-changing event, and you'll need the support of people you love and trust. "It can't be true" is the automatic response for many people, for whom the automatic reaction is one of denial or doubt.

The diagnosis of cancer can often be too much to take in all at once. Cancer is now becoming a treatable long-term condition and many people with cancer will live active and normal lives. Being well-informed about your disease is critical when you receive a diagnosis of bowel cancer. The consequences of your disease will be easier to cope with if you're well-informed, and it'll be easier to make decisions about what to do next.

You will get vital support if you talk to others about your disease, and the situation will become much easier to cope with. The help list at the end of this book contains details of a number of organisations that may come in handy.

Coping with Bowel Cancer after Surgery

Removal of part of the bowel will usually mean that there will be a scar after the operation, especially after open surgery (where the surgeon has made a large incision in the abdomen). A new technique known as laparoscopic surgery (sometimes known as keyhole surgery) is being developed for the removal of bowel cancer. Whilst laparoscopic operations take longer than open surgery, the wounds are very small by comparison and many people who have laparoscopic operations have less pain afterwards and spend less time in hospital.

Blood loss and pain are often issues after open surgery, which is a major procedure with a long recovery time. Embarrassment and self-consciousness can be issues if you end up with a very visible scar. Scarring is less of an issue following keyhole surgery, where the surgeon makes several small incisions between 0.5 and 1.5 cm in length instead of one long, open wound. Surgical instruments can then be passed down a narrow tube called a laparoscope. Through this tube, the tumour can be cut out and removed.

You may be given a blood boosting drug to stop you from suffering the tiredness of anaemia following surgery, while analgesics will be provided to help with the pain. You may require a blood transfusion if the blood loss is significant.

Get some Perspective

Undoubtedly cancer still kills, but our vastly improved knowledge of the disease, coupled with new treatments and screening tests that improve early diagnosis, mean that cancer is now evolving into a manageable long-term condition like diabetes, and people can now live with cancer for many years. For many people, the diagnosis of "cancer" comes completely unexpectedly and this can make the word especially shocking. It's really important that you put the disease into perspective, however.

It's helpful to address the common misconceptions about bowel cancer, as there are plenty of them out there:

"One of my parents or siblings has had bowel cancer. Does this mean I will get it too?"

Whilst there are familial links to bowel cancer, most cases are not genetically linked and the cause is more often unknown, so if one of your first degree relatives as or has had the disease, it doesn't mean that everyone else in the family will get it or even be at a greater risk of getting it. There are no known situations where someone will *definitely* get bowel cancer. Your doctor will be able to find out for definite if you're at risk of developing bowel cancer, and there may be a genetic link if more than one of your first degree relatives has or has had the condition.

"Cancer is a death sentence!"

Cancer treatments have improved dramatically and many cases are being diagnosed earlier. In some cancers including bowel cancer, the disease can be cured if diagnosed very early. Having bowel cancer doesn't necessarily mean you're going to die. Your outcome will be best if it's diagnosed early on so that treatment can be provided. All the same, your life expectancy may not change that much even if you aren't diagnosed straight away, as treatments are now so good that you can live with the condition for many years even without curing it.

"Having had bowel cancer, I feel like half the person I was before."

Nobody will think any less of you because you have or have had cancer. It is very common for people with cancer to give up any hope for the future and for the disease to destroy their confidence and self-esteem. A cancer diagnosis may well change

Cancer treatments have improved dramatically and many cases are being diagnosed earlier. In some cancers including bowel cancer, the disease can be cured if diagnosed very early.

the way you look at things forever, because it's a piece of devastating news. Nobody wants to go through life with cancer on their own, but the vast majority of people will be very supportive when they find out that you have bowel cancer. See the help list for organisations that can help and support you and your family. Remaining active and aiming to live as normal a life as possible will help you to cope with any treatment you might need. Focussing on the positive things in your life like your friends, happy memories and relatives can really boost your confidence, and so can receiving support from others. Always keep in mind that more and more people are surviving cancer, and that surviving this disease is a massive achievement.

"My life will never be the same."

Treatment for early disease can be curative and in this case it can be as if you never had the disease. Even if you have a stoma as part of your treatment, these are very discreet and will not interfere with your daily activities. Just a small scar on your abdomen will be left in most cases, as the majority of stomas are temporary and are eventually removed. It's definitely possible to live a normal life if you've had bowel cancer. While treatment may interfere with your everyday activities and qualities of life, these won't be permanent. The treatment doesn't last forever, and all side effects and problems will disappear over time whether you're receiving chemotherapy, radiotherapy or surgery alone or in combination.

"I have heard that some treatments for cancer such as radiotherapy and chemotherapy can themselves cause new cancers to develop, so isn't it dangerous to have these treatments for bowel cancer?"

People with breast cancer, leukaemia and lymphoma as their primary cancer have developed secondary cancers many years after treatment of their original disease but the rate of secondary cancers is less than 5% in these people. The type of first cancer and treatment will determine whether or not you develop a rare condition known as a secondary malignancy, which is a second cancer that develops after chemotherapy and/or radiotherapy. The benefit of bowel cancer treatment far outweighs the risk, as the risk of getting secondary cancer after treatment for bowel cancer is very low. This is because the form of chemotherapy used for bowel cancer is a lot less aggressive than the form used for breast cancer or leukemia.

"If the treatment is successful and there's no sign of cancer, I must be cured!"

A response to treatment can be defined in many different ways. Unfortunately, true cure is still relatively rare and most people who respond very well to treatment go into remission, which means that there is no evidence of any cancer cells. This is the best possible outcome for most people with cancer and in many cases signs of cancer will not reappear, but a complete remission is not the same as a cure. The reason I mention the difference between cure and remission is that I have heard people being told they are "cured" of cancer only for it to come back many years later (a relapse), with devastating consequences. Stay vigilant. The disease will not come back if you're fully cured, because all of the cancer cells have been destroyed.

I remember a young female work colleague of mine who had been treated for breast cancer with surgery. She was told after her operation that she was cured and didn't need any further treatment. Ten years later she began to get pain in her bones and was feeling continually tired. When she was examined by the local hospital, it was discovered that not only was she not cured, but the cancer had regrown and spread to her bones and liver. Within the next 18 months she had passed away from the disease and left a young family behind. In reality the cancer never really went away in her case and she was not actually cured but in remission and the cancer was still there but undetectable at the time she was told she was cured.

Meanwhile, in remission, the fact that no cancer cells can be detected does not necessarily mean that all of the cancer is gone. Cancer can reappear at some point in the future if the cause is still present after successful treatment, as it often is in cases where bowel cancer arises out of the blue with no identified cause.

If no evidence of cancer can be found in your system, you'll be told you're in complete remission. You have every right to ask your doctor exactly what they mean if they tell you you've been "cured", and finding out whether or not you're really cured can take a lot of time and repeated follow-up visits.

Emotional Support and Counselling

Counselling

Counselling can give you back your hope and a sense of control if you are feeling distressed and powerless to do anything to help yourself. Many people with bowel cancer feel isolated and alone and in these situations counselling and psychotherapy can be very valuable. Talking about bowel cancer with your family and friends may not be something you'll always feel comfortable with. You might worry they'll worry too much once you've told them, or they might be too close or not have enough time. What's more, relatives and friends who know you might not be able to help you understand your situation as well as expressing your feelings and ideas to a professional counselor who doesn't know you might.

After a traumatic or life-changing event, counselling can give you the strength and clear direction you need to carry on. Ignore anyone who suggests that seeing a counsellor (or "shrink") is a sign of weakness.

After a traumatic or life-changing event, counselling can give you the strength and clear direction you need to carry on.

Some years ago I was involved in a serious car crash where my car was hit from behind by another car at high speed on a dual carriageway as I slowed down to pull into a lay-by. My car was hit with such force that it left the road, careened down an embankment and ended up on its roof in a ditch. I was unconscious for several minutes but, remarkably, I was unhurt apart from some scratches and whiplash and was able to crawl out of the car through the back window. Whilst the physical trauma of the crash was minimal the psychological trauma was immense. For weeks afterwards I had recurrent flashbacks and nightmares about the crash and I was terrified of getting back in a car in case the same thing happened again, but I needed a car for my job as a sales rep, so I didn't feel I had any choice but to get back to driving. Fortunately, my employer was very supportive and provided counselling as well as a trained advanced driver to help me get back into the driving seat. The counsellor shared my experience and this was very valuable as my own family were too traumatised themselves to really offer me the support I needed. I also learned some relaxation techniques which stopped the flashbacks and nightmares. Counselling also gave me back the confidence to return to work and have since had more than 10 years of trouble-free driving.

What emotional support is available?

It might be very hard to think positive if you have just been diagnosed with bowel cancer, but this is where emotional support and counselling can really help. Whilst your immediate family and friends might be able to support you, they will not understand what you will be going through in the course of your disease. Despair, anxiety, frustration, loneliness and anger are just a few of the rollercoaster emotions you'll feel while you have cancer.

Your response to treatment and outlook for the future can be negatively affected if these emotions are left uncontrolled and allowed to take over your life. There's nothing wrong with having a good cry if you feel like that's what you need to relieve some of the tension. One of the ways of coping with the knowledge you have cancer is to let go of your emotions.

Many people who have survived bowel cancer have a real desire to give something back and help others with the disease. Talking to other patients with bowel cancer can be a really valuable way of finding people who really get what you're going through. People affected by bowel cancer and their relatives can find support through organisations like Patient Voices, a UK-based patient-to-patient network. More information about Patient Voices can be found in the help list. This group gets involved in funding activities for medical research and charities, supports others through their treatment and raises awareness of the disease.

Life with a Stoma

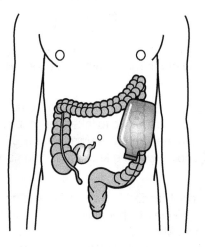

Colostomy
pouch

Stoma fitted with colostomy bag

Having a colostomy can seem like a very distressing lifestyle change and can have a negative effect on your self-esteem, however it is important to remember that many colostomies are only temporary. A stoma will be formed to allow the bowel contents to be emptied outside the body into a stoma bag if you've had an ileostomy or colostomy (see diagram above). Some people learn to flush out their colostomy several times a day and can fit a plug over the stoma instead of using a bag, which can help to build confidence. Most people will be unable to tell you have a colostomy and while it's common to be concerned about the bag smelling or being visible to others, the stoma bags are really very discreet and fit close to the body.

The nurse will provide you with help and education on how to look after your stoma and how to change the bags. In the hospital and at home, trained stoma nurses will be available to support and assist you. If you need further help and support, they will be readily contactable.

Bowel Cancer and Quality of Life

We hardly ever think about quality of life until something happens that affects it in a negative way, often meaning that we can no longer do things as well as we could or cannot do them at all. How well we are able to live our lives and carry out tasks feed in to our estimated quality of life. Your quality of life can be profoundly affected by cancer and its treatment. In extreme cases, the effect of treatment of cancer on quality of life might be so bad that the negative effect on quality of life outweighs any benefit the treatment might deliver. The impact that treatment has can be assessed using a simple tool known as the Linear Analogue Scale Assessment (LASA), a simple scale of 0-100 where 100 represents the best that you can be and 0 represents the worst that you can be (see diagram).

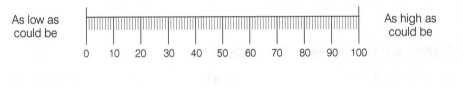

Same scale for:
 energy level
 ability to do daily activities

Linear Analogue Scale Assessment (LASA) for measurement of changes in quality of life

Most healthy people will score themselves between 70-80 on the scale, whereas cancer patients will typically score 30-40. How much of an effect a new treatment has on activities of everyday life is now measured in questionnaires and surveys on quality of life during clinical trials, as the negative effect that diseases such as cancer can have on quality of life is extremely important. When it comes to bowel cancer, treatment will often make quality of life noticeably worse even when the disease itself wasn't having a major impact. When using the LASA scale, patients are asked to mark down how they feel at the time and rate their energy level, ability to carry out activities, and overall quality of life. If it is getting worse, then there are things that can be done to help. The doctor will be able to determine how the quality of life changes if the assessment is repeated at regular intervals throughout treatment. LASA scales and similar assessment tools are becoming a routine part of clinical practice in hospitals around the UK and no longer just during clinical trials, because quality of life in cancer is so important.

Working with Bowel Cancer

A recent change of government legislation offers protection for employees with cancer. This means that employers should not dismiss someone or make them redundant because, for example, they have had extended sick leave for treatment of their cancer, or are unable to do their job as well as before because of the symptoms associated with cancer or its treatment (for example fatigue). Especially if you happen to be the sole or main earner in your family, the ability to keep working during or after bowel cancer treatment is crucial. Employers are not allowed to discriminate against employees with cancer under the Equality Act of 2010. The Macmillan Cancer website has an excellent summary of the Equality Act (details for Macmillan can be found in the help list at the back of this book).

Offering the opportunity to work from home if possible, time off to go to appointments, a gradual return to work after extended sick leave and making alterations to the responsibilities to cater to changing abilities are just a few of the allowances an employer should consider.

Regardless of whether you're working or not, you may be entitled to claim additional financial support, such as the Disability Living Allowance, from the government. The help list at the back of this book includes details on the Directgov website, which holds more information on benefits.

Fatigue from Bowel Cancer

Your ability to do activities of normal daily living, your energy levels and your overall quality of life can be negatively affected by cancer and its treatment. People with diseases, even very common diseases (e.g. a simple flu), can feel extremely fatigued. We tend to think of fatigue in broad terms as a sense of malaise (feeling generally unwell), tiredness, exhaustion or feeling sick.

A simple definition of cancer fatigue is that it is a feeling and a state of tiredness that exceeds the norm, is experienced as clearly unpleasant and does not improve with rest. Healthy people will typically feel exhausted and fatigued after sleep deprivation. Fatigue in people with cancer is a very different concept. Quality of life is damaged especially by fatigue, which is an especially common and debilitating problem in people with cancer. So what's the big deal with cancer-related fatigue? Surely we've all experienced fatigue at some point in our lives! Well, the difference is that a healthy person will recover from their fatigue if they just catch up on their sleep. If they had a flu, they just need to get over the flu and they're over the fatigue. People suffering from other diseases, and healthy people, experience fatigue in a very different way to people with cancer, whose fatigue in relation to their therapy and their tumour is a very different phenomenon.

The disease itself and its treatment can cause fatigue, as can pain and anaemia (these last two can be treated medically and the fatigue is often improved, which in turn improves quality of life). Three cancer treatment centres in Glasgow, Birmingham and Southampton carried out a survey that may give you a better idea of how profoundly cancer-related fatigue can affect people. A total of 576 people with cancer attending outpatient clinics at the treatment centres completed a questionnaire and the results of this survey are dramatic. In 2003, they published their findings. More than half (52%) never discussed fatigue with their doctor and almost half (47%) felt that fatigue was just something they had to put up with. One third of people reported that, unlike pain and nausea/vomiting, the symptoms of their fatigue were poorly controlled. 58% of the people who took part in the survey reported fatigue as a symptom that affected them more than nausea/vomiting, pain or any other reported symptom.

Despite the severity, treatment for fatigue was only offered to 14% of those surveyed. Fatigue can be managed and there are a number of interventions that can help. Here are some comments from people with cancer who suffered from fatigue. This is something we can get a better understanding of if we listen to stories from people who have experienced cancer-related fatigue.

Your ability to do activities of normal daily living, your energy levels and your overall quality of life can be negatively affected by cancer and its treatment.

'Fatigue doesn't just mean being tired. Fatigue is truly the full depression of the body's functions.'

'I have a lot of frustrations and anger over not feeling like doing ordinary things.' 'I was too tired to think . . . '

If you are suffering from fatigue you should always plan your day so that you learn to conserve energy by building in time to rest and do the things that you most want to do – as doing things for yourself is very important. Although resting during the day is important, normal sleep patterns should be maintained, for example waking up at the same time each day. Most importantly, if you feel that you have fatigue and it doesn't get better with rest, talk to your doctor about it.

There appear to be a number of causes for cancer-related fatigue, and the condition is still poorly understood. Especially in cases where the fatigue has been caused or worsened significantly by the treatment, cancer-related fatigue is deeply worrying as it can affect the patient's willingness to continue with their treatment. Fatigue and quality of life can be improved by correcting the anaemia if the person is anaemic and their haemoglobin level is low. Symptoms of fatigue have also been found to be helped by exercise. Sleep can be improved and fatigue decreased if you're able to get regular light exercise. Eating little and often throughout the day can help, drinking plenty of fluids, preparing extra meals when you have the energy. Maintaining your food intake is also important, as a poor diet can cause fatigue.

You can chart whether your fatigue gets better or worse over time if you remember to keep a diary. Showing these records to your doctor can be helpful. If your doctor doesn't know that you have fatigue they cannot help you, and as the results of the survey show this is a trap many people fall into.

What Have We Learned?

- Nobody knows what having cancer is like unless they have had it themselves, but people are very supportive of those with cancer, so it is important to talk to others about your diagnosis.

- Cancer is becoming a treatable, long-term condition and more people are surviving it.

- Having bowel cancer should not prevent you from continuing to work and there is plenty of guidance and support available on this subject.

- Be aware of the difference between remission and cure. A complete remission is almost as good as cure but it is not quite the same thing.

- It is important to put things into perspective, however devastating and upsetting your cancer diagnosis is.

- You will be better able to cope with your condition and any treatment if you're well informed about the process.

- Most stomas are temporary and are very discreet, and you may end up with one if you have surgery to remove part of your bowel.

- If you feel you cannot discuss your disease with the people closest to you, counselling can be very valuable. You may also find a great amount of emotional support from people who have had cancer themselves.

- It is important to talk to your doctor about any negative changes in your quality of life. Some treatment centres actively measure quality of life so they can help you cope, as bowel cancer and its treatment can have a really negative effect.

- Fatigue has the biggest impact on quality of life, and is the most common symptom reported by people with cancer. Some of the causes of fatigue can be managed successfully, so don't lose hope!

8

Further Information

n this chapter, you'll find a list of sources and information on current and future developments into bowel cancer, diagnosis and treatments.

Clinical Trials

ClinicalTrials.gov is an American-based website that lists thousands of clinical research trials being conducted all around the world in a huge variety of diseases including cancer. Cancer Research UK has a clinical trial search page where you can look for clinical trials that are ongoing and recruiting patients. Your doctor may offer you the opportunity to take part in a clinical trial on new treatments or combinations of treatments if your bowel cancer cannot be cured or hasn't responded as well as expected to standard treatment.

People from the UK will often be recruited for trials that are multinational – more information is available at www.clinicaltrials.gov. The website www.cancerhelp.org.uk/trials/ provides information on how to take part in trials, different types of trials and how to find a suitable trial.

Stool DNA Test

This is a noninvasive laboratory test that analyses the cells of a stool sample for changes in DNA. Colon cancer and colon polyps are associated with abnormal DNA which can be identified by the stool DNA test. It's a new method used to screen for colon cancer. Additional testing, such as a colonoscopy to examine the inside of the colon, may be used to investigate the cause if abnormal DNA is detected.

This test can also indicate the presence of cancer by detecting hidden blood in the stool.

Cologuard, a stool DNA test, is approved for colon cancer screening in the United States and UK, though it may only be available in certain hospitals.

More information is available at www.cologuardtest.com.

> Colon cancer and colon polyps are associated with abnormal DNA which can be identified by the stool DNA test.

Oncology Conferences and Symposia

The study of cancer is called oncology. Doctors and other health-care professionals who are involved in the management of bowel cancer often get first access to the latest research data by attending one of the many Oncology Conferences and Symposia that are held around the world.

The ASCO website is often the first place to find the most recent research news on cancer from studies being conducted globally and much of the information on the website is freely available to the public (www.asco.org/). Tens of thousands of oncologists from all over the world attend the ASCO (American Society of Clinical Oncology) each year. It's the largest of the oncology conferences and is held in the USA each May.

A European city hosts the EACR (European Association for Cancer Research) each year, if you're looking for something a little closer to home. The EACR website, www.eacr.org, is a great source for new information on European cancer trials.

EPIC Study (WHO & IARC)

The main findings of the EPIC project so far can be found on the EPIC website, www.epic.iarc.fr/index.php. The EPIC (European Prospective Investigation into Cancer and Nutrition) has been designed to study the incidence of cancer and other chronic diseases in relation to diet, lifestyle, environmental factors and nutritional status. The project has recruited more than 521,000 participants so far, enrolled across 23 centres in 10 western European countries (including the UK). The study began in 1992 and is growing into a long-term project, expected to continue for another number of years.

Glossary

Abdominoperineal resection

A procedure generally carried out for anal or lower rectal cancer. It involves the surgical removal of lymph nodes, the sigmoid colon, rectum and anus and means the patient will need a permanent colostomy.

Accidental Bowel Leakage (fecal incontinence)

Bowel accidents resulting from the inability to retain stool.

Acetaminophen (Tylenol)

A drug that reduces pain and fever, but not inflammation.

Acute

A disease that has a short course but a very rapid onset. The opposite would be "chronic".

Adenocarcinoma

A type of cancerous tumor that can occur in several parts of the body.

Adenoma

A tag of tissue growing in the bowel. See also polyp.

Adhesion

A band of scar tissue that connects two surfaces of the body that are normally separate. This usually happens as a result of surgery or injury.

Adjuvant therapy

Additional cancer treatment given after the primary treatment to lower the risk that the cancer will come back.

Adverse effect

A negative or harmful effect.

Alopecia

Medical term for hair loss.

Anaemia

A condition in which there is a deficiency of red cells or of haemoglobin in the blood, resulting in pallor and weariness.

Analgesic

Medicine to relieve pain.

Anastomosis

In surgery, a procedure that joins two structures, such as reconnecting two ends of the bowel after removal of a section of bowel that contains a tumour.

Antiemetic

A drug that is effective against vomiting and nausea.

Benign

Not cancerous.

Biopsy

A medical procedure that involves taking a small sample of body tissue so it can be examined under a microscope.

BMI (Body Mass Index)
A measure of body mass as a function of body weight divided by the square of the height.

Bolus
The administration of a discrete amount of medication, drug, or other compound within a specific time, generally within 1 - 30 minutes, in order to raise its concentration in blood to an effective level.

Carcinogen
A substance that can cause cancer.

Chronic
A long-term, persistent medical condition or disease, the opposite to "acute".

Colectomy
Surgery to remove part of the colon.

Colonoscopy
A test that uses a narrow, flexible, telescopic camera called a colonoscope to look at the lining of your large bowel.

Constipation
Infrequent bowel movements with stools that are hard and difficult to pass.

Crohn's disease
An inflammatory bowel disease (IBD).

CT scan
Computerised tomography scan which uses X-ray images that are displayed in 3D by computers.

Cure
Recovering from a condition or illness so that it never comes back.

Debulking
In surgery, removing part of a tumour.

Dehydration
This occurs when your body loses more fluid than you take in.

Diabetes
A group of diseases in which the level of sugar in the blood is not properly controlled.

DNA
Short for deoxyribonucleic acid, this is the molecule that contains the genetic code of organisms.

Endocrine
Relating to hormones.

Endoscope
Special flexible tube containing a light and a camera to examine the lining of the GI tract.

Enzyme
Biological catalysts. Substances that speed up chemical reactions without being used up.

Faeces
Another name for waste matter or poo.

Flexible sigmoidoscopy
A procedure that allows your doctor to examine the rectum and the lower (sigmoid) colon.

Gene
A unit of heredity in a living organism, usually a sequence of DNA that produces a protein when it is copied (expressed).

Genetics
The study of genes, genetic variation and heredity in living organisms.

GI

Gastrointestinal.

GP

General Practitioner. This is a doctor who treats people in the wider community, also known as a family doctor.

Gy

Gray – a unit of measurement of radiation dose.

Haem

An iron-containing compound of the porphyrin class which forms the non-protein part of haemoglobin and some other biological molecules.

Haemoglobin

A red-coloured protein containing iron that is found in red blood cells and carries oxygen to the body tissues.

Haemorrhoids

Enlarged blood vessels that you can get inside or around your anus.

Incidence

A measure of the number of new cases of a certain condition, such as cancer, over a defined time period. Usually expressed as a rate (e.g. 50 cases per 1,000 people per year, or 5% per year). Not to be confused with prevalence, which is the total number of cases of a condition in the population at any one time.

Inflammation

A localized physical condition in which part of the body becomes reddened, swollen, hot, and often painful, especially as a reaction to injury or infection.

Infusion

Administration of drugs into a patient through a vein at a steady rate over a period of time.

Inoperable

Not able to be suitably operated on.

Intravenous (IV)

Directly into a vein.

Laxative (purgative, aperient)

A substance that loosens stools and increases bowel movements.

Lymphatic system

A network of vessels in the body that carry tissue fluid (lymph). Part of the immune system.

Malaise

A general feeling of discomfort, illness, or unease whose exact cause is difficult to identify.

Mesentery

A large membrane that surrounds the small and large bowel.

Metastasis

The development of secondary malignant growths at a distance from the primary site of cancer.

MRI scan
Magnetic resonance imaging scans use a strong magnetic field to produce highly detailed images of sections through the body.

Mutation
The permanent alteration of the nucleotide sequence of the genome of an organism, virus or extrachromosomal DNA or other genetic elements.

Nausea
Feeling sick.

Neoadjuvant treatment
Treatment given as a first step to shrink a tumour before the main treatment, which is usually surgery, is given.

Obesity
The condition of being dangerously overweight.

Occult
Not accompanied by readily discernible signs or symptoms.

Oncogene
A gene that has the potential to cause cancer, usually as a result of being mutated or overexpressed.

Oncologist
A doctor who treats cancer and provides medical care for a person diagnosed with cancer.

Oncology
The study of cancer.

Oral
Relating to the mouth.

Palmar-plantar erythema
Redness, soreness and peeling of skin on the hands and feet, a side effect sometimes caused by chemotherapy drugs such as 5-FU.

Polyp
An abnormal growth of tissue projecting from a mucous membrane.

Prevalence
A measure of the total number of cases of a condition such as cancer in the population at any one time. Not to be confused with incidence, which is the number of new cases of the condition.

Prodrug
A medication or compound that, after administration, is metabolised (i.e., converted within the body) into a pharmacologically active drug.

Regimen
A planned course of medical treatment.

Remission
A temporary diminution of the severity of disease or pain.

Screening
In medical terms, a process of trying to identify a disease or condition in people who have no symptoms.

Sedative
Medication prescribed for a sleep-inducing or relaxing effect.

Sensory peripheral neuropathy
A condition that affects sensory nerves causing tingling and/or numbness. A side effect of chemotherapy drugs such as oxaliplatin.

Squamous cell carcinoma
A type of NMSC (non-melanoma skin cancer). The second most common type of skin cancer in the UK.

Staging
A method used by a doctor to determine the size of a tumour and whether it has spread.

Sternum (breastbone)
A long flat bone located in the center of the chest.

Stool
Waste matter (poo) that comes out of your bowels. See also Faeces.

Systemic
Spread throughout, system-wide, affecting a group or system, such as a body.

Tenesmus
A straining sensation in the rectum which can be painful and often results in an inability to pass stools.

Tumour
An abnormal growth of tissue which can be benign or malignant.

Tumour suppressor gene
A gene that can prevent a cell from becoming cancerous.

Ulcerative colitis
A chronic condition where the large intestine (colon and rectum) becomes inflamed.

Vein
Blood vessel that carries blood from the tissues back to the heart.

Vomiting
Emptying the contents of your stomach through your mouth.

Help List

BANT – British Association for Nutrition and Lifestyle Medicine
www.bant.org.uk
Email: theadministrator@bant.org.uk
Post: BANT, 27 Old Gloucester Street, London WC1N 3XX
Telephone: 0870 606 1284
The primary function of BANT is to assist its members in attaining the highest standards of integrity, knowledge, competence and professional practice, in order to protect the client's interests, nutritional therapy and the Nutritional Therapist.

Bowel Cancer UK (previously Beating Bowel Cancer)
www.bowelcanceruk.org.uk
Address: Bowel Cancer UK, Willcox House, 140-148 Borough High Street, London SE1 1LB
Tel: 020 7940 1760
Email: admin@bowelcanceruk.org.uk
UK's leading bowel cancer charity. Provides expert information and support for everyone affected by bowel cancer, and publishes a range of helpful booklets.

British Nutrition Foundation
http://www.nutrition.org.uk/
Address: British Nutrition Foundation, New Derwent House, 69-73 Theobalds Road, London WC1X 8TA.
Tel: 020 7557 7930
Email: postbox@nutrition.org.uk
The British Nutrition Foundation provides nutrition information for teachers, health professionals scientists, and the general public.

British Association for Counselling and Psychotherapy
www.bacp.co.uk
Email: bacp@bacp.co.uk
Phone: 01455 883300
Twitter: @BACP
Post: BACP, 15 St John's Business Park, Lutterworth, Leicestershire LE17 4HB, United Kingdom
This professional association advises schools on setting up counselling services, assists the NHS on service provision, works with voluntary agencies and supports independent practitioners. Find a therapist on their website.

Cancer Research UK

www.cancerresearchuk.org/

Address: Angel Building, 407 St John Street, London, EC1V 4AD

Tel: 0300 123 1022

Email: supporter.services@cancer.org.uk

Funds scientists, doctors and nurses to help beat cancer sooner. Provides cancer information to the public.

Department of Health and Social Care

www.gov.uk/dh

Address: Ministerial Correspondence and Public Enquiries Unit, Department of Health and Social Care, 39 Victoria Street, London SW1H 0EU, United Kingdom

Tel: 020 7210 4850

A ministerial department supporting ministers in leading the nation's health and social care to help people live more independent, healthier lives for longer.

Food & Drink Federation

www.fdf.org.uk/

Address: 6th Floor, 10 Bloomsbury Way, London WC1A 2SL

Tel: 020 7836 2460

The voice of the UK food and drink industry, which is the largest manufacturing sector in the country.

GOV.UK

www.gov.uk

This is a government website that provides useful information on benefits and financial support for those with long-term conditions such as cancer. Contact details for services local to you can be found through the website.

Macmillan Cancer Support

www.macmillan.org.uk

Address: 89 Albert Embankment, London, SE1 7UQ

Tel: 0808 808 00 00

Macmillan Cancer Support is a voluntary organisation that provides practical, medical and financial support for people living with cancer. Macmillan has a national presence so you should be able to find help and support close to you. The website has a huge amount of useful information on all aspects of cancer.

National Institute for Health and Care Excellence

https://cks.nice.org.uk/bowel-screening

Address: 10 Spring Gardens, London SW1A 2BU

Manchester: Level 1A, City Tower, Piccadilly Plaza, Manchester M1 4BT

Tel: +44 (0)300 323 0140

The National Institute for Health and Care Excellence (NICE) provides national guidance and advice to improve health and social care.

NHS Bowel Cancer Screening (BCSP) Programme

https://www.gov.uk/topic/population-screening-programmes/bowel

Address: Public information access office, Public Health England, Wellington House, 133-155 Waterloo Road, London SE1 8UG, United Kingdom

Tel: 020 7654 8000

List of information about NHS bowel cancer screening (BCSP) programme.

NHS Change4Life

www.nhs.uk/change4life

Tel: 0300 123 4567

The NHS Change4Life website was designed to encourage adults and children to get fit and active, eating well, moving more and living longer as a result.

The website contains lots of tips and useful information on healthy eating and exercise. It is a good way of finding activities in your local area that you might wish to join.

NHS Choices

www.nhs.uk/conditions/Cancer-of-the-colon-rectum-or-bowel/Pages/Introduction.aspx

A great source of information about bowel cancer symptoms, causes, treatment and diagnosis.

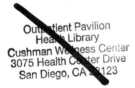

CPSIA information can be obtained
at www.ICGtesting.com
Printed in the USA
LVHW101359131220
674072LV00007B/417